Trauma, Women's Mental Health, and Social Justice

This book argues that while notions of trauma in mental health hold promise for the advancement of women's rights, the mainstreaming of trauma treatments and therapies has had mixed implications, sometimes replacing genuine social change efforts with new forms of female oppression by psychiatry. It contends that trauma interventions often represent a "business as usual" approach within psychiatry, with women being expected to comply with rigid treatment protocols, accepting the advice given by trauma "experts" that they are mentally unstable and that they must learn to manage the effects of violence in the absence of any real changes to their circumstances or resources. A critique of trauma treatment in its current form, *Trauma, Women's Mental Health, and Social Justice* recommends practical steps towards a socio-political perspective on trauma which passionately re-engages with feminist values and activist principles.

Emma Tseris is a Lecturer in Social Work and Policy Studies at the University of Sydney, Australia, where her research and teaching areas include critical mental health theory, mental health and gender inequality, and narrative research methodologies.

Routledge Research in Gender and Society

For more information about this series, please visit: www.routledge.com/sociology/series/SE0271

Trauma, Women's Mental Health, and Social Justice

Pitfalls and Possibilities

Emma Tseris

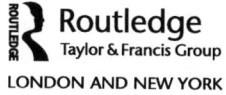
Routledge
Taylor & Francis Group

LONDON AND NEW YORK

First published 2019
by Routledge
2 Park Square, Milton Park, Abingdon, Oxon OX14 4RN

and by Routledge
52 Vanderbilt Avenue, New York, NY 10017

First issued in paperback 2020

Routledge is an imprint of the Taylor & Francis Group, an informa business

© 2019 Emma Tseris

The right of Emma Tseris to be identified as author of this work has been asserted by her in accordance with sections 77 and 78 of the Copyright, Designs and Patents Act 1988.

British Library Cataloguing-in-Publication Data
A catalogue record for this book is available from the British Library

Library of Congress Cataloging-in-Publication Data
Names: Tseris, Emma, author.
Title: Trauma, women's mental health, and social justice : pitfalls and possibilities / Emma Tseris.
Description: Abingdon, Oxon ; New York, NY : Routledge, 2019. | Series: Routledge research in gender and society ; 77 | Includes bibliographical references and index.
Identifiers: LCCN 2018055750 (print) | LCCN 2018058920 (ebook) | ISBN 9781315107820 (eBook) | ISBN 9781138091801 (hardback) | ISBN 9781315107820 (ebk)
Subjects: | MESH: Psychological Trauma | Women's Health—trends | Social Justice | Feminism
Classification: LCC RG103.5 (ebook) | LCC RG103.5 (print) | NLM WM 172.5 | DDC 616.890082—dc23
LC record available at https://lccn.loc.gov/2018055750

ISBN 13: 978-0-367-66027-7 (pbk)
ISBN 13: 978-1-138-10380-1 (hbk)

Typeset in Times New Roman
by Apex CoVantage, LLC

This book is dedicated to the many courageous and intelligent women who have shared their knowledge with me over the past few years, whether in a research interview or a less formal conversation, in order that I might see the silences, flaws, and ongoing limitations within the frameworks that have been positioned as "best practice" in mental health. I hope that this book captures some of your hopes about the broad system changes required in order for justice to become possible.

I wish to acknowledge the traditional owners of the land on which I work and live, the Gadigal people of the Eora Nation; to recognise the invaluable contributions of Aboriginal and Torres Strait Islander knowledges relating to social and emotional wellbeing; and to pay respect to Aboriginal and Torres Strait Elders past, present, and emerging.

Contents

Preface

Despite compelling critiques of patriarchal power and the emergence of incisive strategies to address gender inequality in contemporary times – the #MeToo movement being a prominent example that emerged during the writing of this book – we nonetheless continue to live in perilous times for women and children. The multitude of social developments made possible by feminist thinking continue to face almost constant backlash, as feminist concerns are simultaneously trivialised and de-politicised (Benton-Grieg, Gamage, & Gavey, 2018). On the other side of this argument, of course, sits the notion that feminism has always faced hostility; its demands have persistently drawn into question the existing order of things, and consequently its future has always been precarious and uncertain. Keeping these contestations in mind, within this book feminist theory is utilised as a framework to critically explore the contemporary shift within mental health discourses towards accounting for and responding to the effects of gender-based violence on mental wellbeing. Looking specifically at the consequences of the emergence and growth of the trauma paradigm as a way of making sense of mental distress, the book aims to explore how the experiences of women who come to the attention of psychiatric services, either during or following exposure to gender-based violence, are shaped by trauma discourses. In doing so, it offers an analysis of both the transformative and empowering capacity of trauma-informed practices, as well as their potentially delimiting and oppressive implications for women.

In the past two decades, numerous books on the usefulness of trauma principles within mental health services have become available. While *Trauma, Women's Mental Health, and Social Justice* will cover some familiar territory for the readers of such titles, it offers a different analysis to the majority of the available literature on trauma: through utilising the lenses of critical mental health theory and feminist analysis, it provides an in-depth exploration of the notion that the contemporary use of the trauma paradigm within mental health services is connected to a progressive social justice project. Its overarching aim is to explore the social and political consequences of the increasing prominence of the trauma paradigm as a guiding framework within mental health services. In doing this work, the book engages critically with the widespread assumption that trauma-informed practices are inherently or necessarily aligned to feminist aims, and in turn, the empowerment of women within mental health settings. Throughout its analysis, the book attempts to consider the real-world implications of the trauma paradigm on the lives of women who come to the attention of mental health services. In particular, the book explores how trauma-informed ideas and practices have, in the past quarter of a century, moved from marginal to mainstream concepts informing mental health service provision, and it considers the array of potential consequences of this shift for women accessing mental health and therapeutic support. Thank you for picking up this book and engaging with these concerns, which I hope that we can start to examine collectively. Please be in touch if you would like to share some ideas or responses. It would be wonderful to start to think together about some creative ways to engage in conversations about trauma, violence, gender, mental health, and social justice.

Reference

Benton-Greig, P., Gamage, D., & Gavey, N. (2018). Doing and denying sexism: Online responses to a New Zealand feminist campaign against sexist advertising. *Feminist Media Studies*, *18*(3), 349–365.

Acknowledgements

To each of the participants who shared their knowledge and experiences with me, I am immensely grateful for your time and expertise – thank you. I would like to express my sincere gratitude to Associate Professor Lesley Laing and Associate Professor Margot Rawsthorne, for providing a perfect combination of commitment, positivity, intelligence, and humour during my PhD candidature and in the years following, and to Professor Sue Goodwin, for research mentorship. Thanks also to Dr Bruce Cohen, for your tremendous encouragement and collegiality, and of course, your inspiring work in critical mental health theory. Thank you to Amelia Boyers for your excellent research assistance relating to the nexus between trauma, neuroscience, and attachment theory. I would like to also extend my gratitude to Neil Jordan at Routledge, for believing that the issues that I have been wrestling with over these past few years are worth putting together in this book. Of course, none of this would have been possible without my family and friends – thank you for all of the unseen support. Finally, I would like to thank Rhys, for your love and for your kindness, and for always being so obliging during the many hours that we have spent talking through the intricate and sometimes obscure details of trauma discourses.

List of abbreviations

APA	American Psychiatric Association
BPD	Borderline Personality Disorder
BTQ	Brief Trauma Questionnaire
CBT	Cognitive Behavioural Therapy
C-PTSD	Complex Post-Traumatic Stress Disorder
DBT	Dialectical Behavioural Therapy
DSM	Diagnostic and Statistical Manual of Mental Disorders
ECT	Electroconvulsive Therapy
EMDR	Eye Movement Desensitisation and Reprocessing
ICD	International Classification of Diseases
PTSD	Post-Traumatic Stress Disorder

1 Introducing a critical perspective on trauma

A "trauma-informed" approach to understanding people experiencing mental distress has – in the space of a couple of decades – moved from being a little-known, activist notion, to a paradigm that has been eagerly embraced within mental health services. Though not inevitable, trauma is viewed as a common and understandable response to violence and a range of other overwhelming experiences, and the concept of trauma has garnered mounting influence within human service practice, policy, research, and education contexts. Far from its original positioning as a peripheral concept, contemporary mental health policy documents, funding proposals, and service delivery statements are now imbued with notions of "trauma-informed care". The turn towards trauma has been described as offering "a 'new generation' of transformed mental health and human service organisations and programs" (Bateman, Henderson, & Kezelman, 2013, p. 4), and the vast majority of scholarship on trauma-informed practices has taken a highly optimistic view of its benefits – particularly in terms of its capacity to offer a compassionate and contextualised perspective on mental health presentations, through its consideration of the life events that may lead to mental distress. Trauma-informed practices are routinely compared favourably in comparison to conventional mental health service provision. While the latter emphasises the assessment and management of symptoms, trauma work – it is argued – allows for a socio-contextual analysis of the origins of emotional distress. This book differs in the analysis that it offers relating to trauma-informed mental health services, providing a more careful reading of the trauma paradigm, and examining in particular its implications for women (while acknowledging that trauma discourses also hold many implications for other individuals and communities, including refugees and asylum seekers, people experiencing poverty, and people experiencing various forms of violence and discrimination other than or in addition to gendered oppressions). While there have been extensive medical and psychological investigations into trauma that have examined its causes, treatments, and the possibility of recovery, there has been limited critical analysis that has situated trauma as a socially constructed concept, allowing for an exploration of its underlying assumptions and relations of power.

While trauma-informed practices are used rather broadly within mental health services, thus affecting a wide range of mental health service users, this book contends that turning a spotlight onto women's experiences of the trauma paradigm is a valid focus. The psychiatric profession has a very long history of disproportionately labelling women as mentally ill, leading to a range of mental health interventions specifically designed to control and manage women's perceived mental dysfunctions – a bias that continues to this day (Ussher, 2011). In addition, a significant amount of attention within trauma literature centres on the effects of rape, domestic violence, and child sexual assault – experiences that are clearly gendered due to women and girls being so disproportionately affected (Moulding, 2015). When considering the turn to trauma within mental health policy and service provision contexts, women as a group have been particularly affected; for example, trauma-informed therapeutic support is often recommended as a "best practice" response to women when experiences of sexual assault and other gender-based violence have been disclosed. This is an important shift: after decades of ignoring women's social experiences, and viewing mental and emotional distress as arising due to purely biological processes, ideas about the importance of negative life events in shaping women's lives are becoming increasingly more widely accepted within psychiatric settings. Rosenthal, Reinhardt, and Birrell (2016) note that a "trauma-informed" approach is underpinned by a number of assumptions:

- Human experiences of an overwhelming or devastating nature leave predictable and understandable marks on survivors' minds and bodies.
- While mainstream mental health services have usually viewed such difficulties as mental health disorders, they should instead be seen as causally linked to the events that have occurred.
- When the connection between events and distress is not made, mental health service users are pathologised by the mental health system, as they are seen as "disordered" individuals, while their social contexts are ignored.

It is this book's contention that the trauma paradigm's construction of an "experience-distress" nexus has both liberating and troubling implications for women who come to the attention of mental health services. This book enthusiastically concurs with Becker-Blease's (2017, p. 131) claim that while the trauma paradigm without doubt carries much emancipatory potential for women, we must start to "critically engage with the devils in the details" – a task that has become especially urgent given the exponential rise in the popularity of the term "trauma-informed". While acknowledging the conceptual and practical improvements that trauma discourses have made to the traditional diagnostic model of mental health is important, it is also crucial for mental health workers and researchers who are knowledgeable about the limitations of biological explanations of mental distress to subject any new-found certainties about the causes of distress to critical analysis. Within this age of biomedical psychiatry, it is a refreshing reprieve to come across ideas that are less reductionist or deterministic than those provided by the medical model of mental illness. Nevertheless, it is the stance taken in this book that ideas about the social factors underpinning distress, and the efficacy of therapeutic (as opposed

to medical) responses, are not immune from political biases or professional interests. Moreover, the need for critical analysis exists regardless of whether one's
professional training is inside or outside of psychiatry (for example, in sociology,
social work, nursing, psychology, or art therapy), and it remains relevant even if
a mental health treatment modality is open to accepting socio-contextual explanations of mental distress.

Unfortunately, once conversations about mental health shift from biomedical topics towards an engagement with "social" or biographical factors and their
effects, there is often an inherent assumption that the analysis that is being offered
is benevolent and free from power relations or biases. Frequently, such analyses
interrogate the fallibilities of psychopharmacology, and call for a rise in the number of talking professionals or therapists (for example, Gnaulati, 2018). As will be
explored throughout this book, however, therapy is not an innocent endeavour –
even if a staunch anti-medication stance is taken, or if the approach used by a
worker is to develop an explicitly "collaborative" partnership with service users,
or if the work is shaped by a trauma-informed perspective. Rather, therapeutic
work is deeply embedded in cultural, socio-political, and gendered processes,
and such processes are not neutral. Thus, trauma-informed therapeutic practices
should be subjected to sociological critique. As noted by feminist anti-psychiatry
academic, Burstow (2018), any position that is formulated within the constraints
of mental health discourses – however progressive its intentions – is compro-
mised by the ongoing constraints of a mental health focus on locating dysfunctions within service users. Such discourses are shaped by notions of individual
pathology and the assumption that distress is solvable through a combination of
professional interventions and self-help efforts.

Importantly, in providing a critical perspective on trauma-informed practices,
the intention of this book is not to undermine the feminist efforts that have led
to the development of trauma-informed practices within mental health services,
nor to deny the improvements that trauma-informed practices have made possible. Rather, this book has emerged out of a concern that at times the trauma
paradigm is being positioned as having resolved the inadequacies of a psychiatric
explanation of distress (particularly women's distress), leading to an inability to
fully examine the socio-political implications of the turn to trauma within mental
health services. It also attempts to address the question of whether the feminist
underpinnings of the trauma paradigm can retain their influence as trauma discourses are utilised within mainstream mental health services. Therefore, it is
not the intention of the book to assume a position of lofty theorising, in which
the limitations of current mental health practices are determined, without offering any useful alternatives. Worse still, I do not wish to overlook the multitude
of ways in which feminists working within the walls of mental health services
have tirelessly advocated for a system that not only acknowledges women's
experiences, but that highlights gender inequality and gender-based violence as
fundamental to the assessment of women's mental health presentations. Trauma-
informed practices have been an important, and at times, central component of
these feminist efforts.

The perceived gap that exists between the research world and the world of human service practice is a critique of the role of academic work that I have reflected upon while writing this book, and I have attempted to avoid the perceived limitations of academic contributions to mental health practice in a number of ways. Firstly, my analysis of trauma-informed practices has been inspired by both informal conversations and formal interviews with mental health service users over the period I have been involved in research (and prior to this as a mental health social worker), who have shared with me their concerns about contemporary mental health provision, their experiences of psychiatric harm, and their ideas about alternative responses to people experiencing distress. In Chapter 5, I report on a research study involving in-depth interviews with women survivors of gender-based violence and their exposure to mental health and therapeutic support. The power differential that exists between mental health service users and workers means that it is usually extremely difficult, and often unsafe for mental health service users to offer a critique or to protest against contemporary service provision. My privileged position enables me to much more freely articulate a critique and to provide a counter-narrative, although it brings up a vast array of difficult questions about how this work might be approached in an ethical manner – for example, it is important that I acknowledge that my name as the sole author of this book invisibilises the expertise of others. Secondly, my ideas have been shaped by numerous discussions with critically minded mental health workers, who have shared with me their understandings of the possibilities and potential limits of trauma-informed practices. Chapter 4's exploration of the relationships between neuroscience, attachment theory, and trauma discourses came about as a result of conversations with feminist mental health workers expressing their hesitations about the under-examined implications of the turn towards trauma, and their concerns that trauma-informed practices alone cannot be seen as a solution to the individualising effects of the biological framing of mental distress.

Key concepts and debates in the book

The understanding of feminism that is used within this book is that it is a heterogeneous movement, with diverse voices and perspectives, giving rise to lively and useful debates and contestations. At its core, however, "feminism is a movement to end sexism, sexist exploitation and oppression" (hooks, 2000, p. viii). In line with a feminist analysis, gender-based violence is defined as violence against women and children that is specifically constructed by the power relations of hetero-patriarchy (Radford, Kelly, & Hester, 1996). This understanding is grounded in the work of second-wave feminists, who worked tirelessly to generate public awareness about the prevalence of domestic violence, sexual assault, and child abuse, highlighting the deleterious effects of these experiences on women and children. Feminist activism facilitated an awareness of how such experiences are bound by systemic practices of male power and privilege (Reid, 2018), with some women experiencing multiple forms of violence throughout their lifecourse (Cleary & Hungerford, 2015). While not ignoring women's use of violence, feminist analysis demonstrated that such violence differs in frequency, severity, and intention (Kimmel, 2002). Furthermore, it established that when men are victims of violence, the perpetrator is most often male (Taft, Hegarty, & Flood, 2001); it critiqued pervasive practices of mother-blaming in relation to male-perpetrated violence (Moulding, Buchanan, & Wendt, 2015); and it eluci-dated the need for maternal violence against children to be viewed in terms of its interaction with co-occurring intimate partner violence (Namy et al., 2017).

Third-wave and intersectional feminism expanded on the work of second-wave feminism by attempting to redress the elevation of particular voices and expe-riences within the women's liberation movement (those of white, middle class, able-bodied, cisgender women) at the expense of others. This analysis showed the ways in which feminism was involved in side-lining the experiences of women in some of the most marginalised social locations, while pursuing the agendas of women who already enjoy larger social privileges and resources (Thiara & Gill, 2010). More contemporary perspectives are demonstrating the ways in which the women's movement has been affected by the neoliberal turn towards individual-ism and consumption, neglecting its roots as a social movement based on col-lectivism, with an awareness of the importance of social policy and community change rather than personal aspiration. These failings have led to some people rejecting feminism outright (Crispin, 2017). However, others, such as Roxanne Gay (2014) have argued that while feminism must improve its intersectional analysis of diverse women's lives, expecting feminism to completely avoid these pitfalls means holding feminism to a higher standard than any other social justice movement. It is important, Gay contends, to avoid conflating the failings and biases of *people* with the failings of *feminism*. The approach taken in this book is that the multiple contributions of feminist theories provide a crucial framework to analyse the meanings of trauma perspectives in mental health, and to critically explore their consequences. In developing this analysis, feminist theory is used in conjunction with the tools of poststructuralism and critical mental health theory, which are outlined in Chapter 2.

The term "discourses" is used within the book to refer to the myriad ways in which people act upon and make meaning within the social world: "discourses are more than language – they are ways of behaving, interacting, valuing, think-ing, believing, speaking – discourses are 'ways of being in the world'" (Locke, 2004, p. 7). Despite there being a variety of discourses available within the social world, certain discourses are more dominant and influential than others. Pow-erful groups have excessive capacities to perpetuate their views of the world, resulting in the propagation of dominant discourses, leading to the most power-ful knowledges with the largest "subscription" base becoming *hegemonic* dis-courses (Locke, 2004). Meanwhile, the "local" understandings of marginalised groups become "disqualified" knowledges, and are treated as though they lack legitimacy (Foucault, 1980). For example, mental health discourses (the practices, language, concepts, and understandings of the mental health professions) are cur-rently the dominant means through which a large proportion of human problems are understood, leading to other explanations of human experience being rendered invisible. In this way, notions of mental health and mental illness can be viewed as socially constructed – while the existence of human suffering and "madness" is not in dispute, medical understandings are culturally and historically situated knowledges, which are therefore open to contestation. Within the book, I use the term *trauma discourses* in order to argue that the "taken-for-granted" status that is often afforded to trauma and trauma-informed practices within mental health settings is problematic. In other words, trauma should not be viewed as an objective concept, but rather as a paradigm that has arisen within particular socio-political and professional contexts, which has been informed by a number of assumptions that should be viewed with a critical analysis – for example, ideas about the centrality of therapeutic mental health interventions after violence. This is not the same as arguing that trauma and trauma-informed practices have never been helpful for women; rather, while the concept of trauma is helpful in some circumstances, this book argues that its utilisation at other times is hazardous and limiting; that claims about its universal relevance are unwarranted; and that caution is required as the trauma concept gains more and more traction within mental health settings.

The terms "trauma-informed practices", the "trauma concept", and "trauma paradigm" are used to refer to the broad – and increasingly contested – bod(ies) of knowledge that explore the effects of a range of adverse life experiences on mental wellbeing across the lifecourse. Trauma is defined within mainstream mental health settings as the psychological effects of exposure to actual or threatened death, serious injury, or sexual violation (American Psychiatric Association, 2013), with some authors advocating for a broader definition that can incorporate additional experiences, for example emotional abuse, which are not life-threatening but are frequently humiliating and oppressive (Briere & Scott, 2015). Another significant contestation relating to definitions of trauma is that the term trauma is not only used to describe the psychological *effects* of particular events, but it is also commonly used to describe overwhelming events or stressors themselves – for example, "the trauma [event] has caused a trauma [reaction]". Consequently, an unhelpful elision has emerged, with trauma sometimes being used to describe both an event and its effects (Gilfus, 1999). This overlapping usage is confusing, and it unhelpfully contributes to the notion that adverse events and trauma are inevitably connected. It also means that "trauma" is sometimes used as a euphemism or replacement word for violence, which has de-politicising effects (Tseris, 2018). Within this book, then, care is taken to separate acts of violence from ideas about their negative and long-lasting effects. To do this, I have avoided using the term "trauma" or "traumatic event" when referring to experiences of violence or abuse, using it only when discussing the potential effects of such experiences (although participant quotations in the research findings presented in Chapter 5 remain unedited, as are the direct quotations of research that are analysed throughout the book).

Crucially, challenging the contemporary status afforded to trauma discourses is not the same as minimising or disbelieving women's stories of abuse or ignoring women's own understandings of the effects of gender-based oppressions on their lives, nor is it analogous to ignoring harm or distress. Rather, a critical perspective on trauma argues that it is the variety of assumptions that have clustered around experiences of gender-based oppressions that are in need of critique, for example, universalising notions of the effects of such violations, as well as prescriptive professional narratives that provide only a very narrow set of therapeutic responses after violence. Indeed, it is this book's contention that a critical analysis of the trauma paradigm is not about minimising violence and its effects; rather, critical thinking is aimed at re-asserting the importance of survivors' voices and knowledges, and demonstrating the ways in which some iterations of the trauma concept are involved in covering up complexities, promoting professional agenda, and reducing the range of experiences and responses that are able to be considered.

Trauma-informed services have sometimes been differentiated from trauma therapies, with the former referring to a broad paradigm being rolled out across all segments of human service provision that acknowledges that many service users have experienced traumatic life events, and attempts to provide a context that is sensitive to these histories (for example, through notions of collaboration, transparency, safety, and changes to the physical environment), while the latter specifically develops "treatments" for the effects of trauma (Sweeney, Clement, Filson, & Kennedy, 2016). Although this distinction is useful, as some human service systems aim to adhere to trauma-informed principles while not engaging with the specific experiences of service users, many of the aims of a generic and a treatment-focused understanding of trauma are similar: although not directly addressing past experiences, trauma-informed services aim to view the presenting issues of service users as arising within a context of exposure to violence or other overwhelming experiences (Levenson, 2017). The two approaches are linked, in that a generic trauma-informed approach includes the use of referral pathways to therapeutic services for trauma-based interventions (NSW Kids and Families, 2014). Further, this book is focused on trauma discourses within mental health settings, and mental health services are nearly always concerned with offering treatments or responses at the level of individuals. Mental health service users are likely to be affected both by broad policy directions towards trauma-informed service provision, as well as the enactment of trauma discourses within therapeutic encounters aimed at addressing their mental health presentations. Another distinction is sometimes made between "acute" and "complex" trauma, to distinguish between the effects of a single overwhelming event as opposed to the effects of ongoing interpersonal abuse, perpetrated by a known person (Bath, 2008). The latter is characteristic of a large proportion – though not all – forms of gender-based violence, and some trauma-informed therapies have been constructed to address "complex" trauma specifically. Contestations about what should "count" as trauma, how trauma is defined, and with what implications are explored further in Chapters 3, 4, and 6.

"Psychocentrism", and "psychiatric hegemony", are terms that refer to the pervasive outlook within contemporary Western societies that all human problems can be traced to individual pathologies of the mind and/or brain (Rimke & Brock, 2012). Psychiatric hegemony refers to the pervasive view that emotional distress is a medical issue that can be categorised into one or a number of psychiatric "disorders". Its positioning as a grand (hegemonic) narrative has resulted in an abundance of mental health professionals and an ever-increasing number of psychiatric illnesses in the *Diagnostic and Statistical Manual of Mental Disorders* (DSM), a publication of the American Psychiatric Association (APA), now in its fifth edition. While psychiatric discourses refer to a diagnostic and medication approach to treating mental illness, psychocentrism refers to the high status afforded to psychological or therapeutic understandings within contemporary societies, which also focus on dysfunctions within individuals, but emphasise management strategies including formal therapy, emotion management, and self-help (Anderson, Brownlie, & Given, 2009). In the past couple of decades, there has been a sharp rise in literature that has focused on deconstructing psychiatric knowledges and positioning therapeutic practices as the solution to the narrow scope and dehumanising effects of psychiatry (for example, Bentall, 2010). In contrast to the notion that psychiatric and psychological/therapeutic practices are diametrically opposed, this book takes the view that psychiatric and therapeutic discourses are often informed by similar assumptions, and therefore share similar limitations. For example, both psychiatric and therapeutic approaches to human distress frequently interpret experiences in ways that invisibilise socio-political issues, by identifying dysfunctions within individuals. This point is an important component of the critique of the trauma paradigm that is offered within the following chapters. Although the trauma concept advocates the use of therapy as an alternative to medication and diagnosis, it has often failed to examine broader opportunities for social change and feminist activism regarding violence against women, continuing instead to focus on the mental states of individual women.

Following Rose's (1998) use of the terms "psy-professions" and "psy-complex" to refer to the set of professions and professional approaches that have been set up to attend to issues pertaining to human behaviour and mental states, the terms "mental health workers" and "mental health interventions" are used broadly in this book, to refer to the broad range of professional disciplines and knowledges that are charged with the roles of addressing and regulating mental health and illness. Although this book locates psychiatry as the most dominant mental health profession, it is interested in exploring how the mental health professions as a whole are engaged in responding to people who have been categorised with a mental difference (whether this difference is deemed to be mental illness, a trauma reaction, or a combination of the two). In reality, although psychiatrists are the principle mental health professionals involved in diagnostic and assessment processes, mental health professionals across disciplinary divides draw upon the Diagnostic and Statistical Manual of Mental Disorders (DSM) – if not formally, by utilising its ideas and assumptions more generally (Lacasse, 2014), and mental health professionals from a variety of disciplines have become involved in trauma therapies and trauma-informed practices. Importantly, this book does not set out to criticise mental health workers as individuals, although it does suggest that mental health workers could benefit from enhanced reflexivity about their work, the social status of the psy-professions, and the assumptions upon which psychiatric and therapeutic discourses are built.

This book follows social and critical perspectives on mental health, and where possible replaces the term "mental illness" with "distress" – while keeping in mind that "distress" is also too narrow to incorporate the experiences of all people who come to the attention of mental health services, and is a term that may continue to invite the unwanted interventions of medical and therapeutic professionals in search of a cure, as well as contributing to the perceived passivity of service users. The book conceptualises "mental illness" as a widespread – yet limited and contestable – descriptor of emotional distress and difference. In drawing on the work of critical mental health scholars, the book draws upon work that uses the term "madness" as an alternative phrase for mental illness. "Madness" is a reclaimed term used by some mental health activists as a means of defining their own experiences outside of dominant professional and community discourses. It offers a much less prescriptive concept than mental illness, to the point of being almost deliberately vague in order to incorporate a vast range of unusual or distressing human experiences and perceptions, without resorting to an unhelpful dichotomy between "normality" and "abnormality".

As the term "social justice" has become an overused and under-explored "catchphrase" within recent decades (North, 2006), it is worthwhile to outline its use within this book. Social justice theorising has tended to focus on a re-distributive justice paradigm, based upon a fair distribution of resources across society, however in the area of mental health there are further social justice questions that require investigation (Josewski, 2017). For example, critical mental health writers have demonstrated that re-distribution aims are insufficient in addressing the pervasive exclusion and symbolic violence experienced by people labelled as mentally ill, and the silencing of their voices across research and policy contexts (Liegghio, 2013; Poole et al., 2012). Furthermore, there is a need to interrogate the social construction of mental illness, and to critique the positioning of "mental illness" as an objective entity – while at the same time, continuing to attend to serious material concerns affecting people labelled as mentally ill. Therefore, it is the contention of this book that social justice questions in the area of mental health must be interested in "social arrangements that can redress both economic and cultural injustices" (Fraser, 2009, p. 86).

Finally, I have decided to use the term "service user" to refer to people who come into contact with mental health services. McLaughlin (2008) explored the changing language used to describe those who receive services by human service professionals ("patient", "client", "customer", "consumer", "expert by experience", "service user"), without providing an easy answer as to the most ideal term. The term "patient" is clearly problematic as it is imbued with notions of pathology and passivity, and constructs mental illness as indistinguishable from physical illness. "Consumer" and "customer" are meanwhile infused with notions of a marketised relationship, whereby those receiving mental health services are positioned as in control of what occurs – a construction of the professional relationship that often ignores an experience of disempowerment, indignity, or lack of autonomy. While the newer term "expert by experience" is a refreshing attempt to transform negative and deficit-laden assumptions about those receiving services – re-positioning them as highly knowledgeable and able to provide useful critiques of the weaknesses of service systems – it is also an overly vague term. It places all people who have received services into one category, ignoring their highly diverse experiences and perceptions of these services. Also, the homogenisation of "lived experience" invisibilises the range of expertise that any one person may have, often from multiple sources beyond the personal and experiential, or the common scenario of a "dual identity", whereby a person may be a mental health worker who has at some point been a service user. "Psychiatric survivor" is the most politicised term available to describe people who have received psychiatric attention. Despite the obvious benefits of this term, it is unable to incorporate the experiences of people who report that the mental health support that they have received has been voluntary, useful or with mixed benefits. For these reasons, although "service user" is not a perfect term, it is one of the broadest and least pathologising among those in regular use and it is inclusive of people who have found mental health services useful and those who have not, as well as people who have chosen to use mental health services and people who have not consented to mental health interventions.

Outline of the book

Having outlined in this chapter an introductory justification for the need for the development of a critical perspective on trauma, Chapter 2 looks at the limitations of contemporary mental health discourses more broadly. It explores the ways in which mental health discourses are deeply implicated in perpetuating dominant societal values and relations of power, for example, patriarchal power relations and neoliberalism. Key elements of critical mental health theory and feminist analyses are discussed in terms of the contributions that they have made to understanding how psychiatric discourses are implicated in perpetuating gendered oppressions and other forms of social inequality. The chapter then explores the contributions made by third-wave and intersectional feminist analyses, which allow for more nuanced accounts of women's engagement with psychiatric discourses than is possible within a representation of straightforward oppression. For example, such analyses explore differences among women in their experiences of psychiatry, as well as allowing space for a consideration of how women engage strategically in acts of resistance against psychiatric claims.

Chapter 3 then specifically analyses the rising use of trauma-informed discourses within contemporary mental health settings, examining the ways in which the trauma paradigm is thought to circumvent the many limitations of biomedical psychiatry and lead to services that are informed by feminist understandings. It discusses the potential benefits of trauma-informed practices for women, including the long-overdue recognition of women's social contexts and experiences. However, it also discusses numerous cautions relating to the transformative capacities of the trauma paradigm. Too often, trauma-informed discourses remain invested in the conventional aims of symptom assessment and individual treatment, and notions of a linear trajectory between experiences of violence and psychological harm. Chapter 4 continues the critical analysis of trauma discourses by exploring the use of neuroscience data to bolster the claims of trauma-informed practices, as well as the burgeoning research area investigating the nexus between violence, abuse, and mothering capacity. Troublingly, such contemporary directions in trauma research suggest a distancing of the trauma paradigm from its espoused connection to women's empowerment and a critique of patriarchal power. This chapter concludes by examining how the amorphous nature of the trauma paradigm leaves it open to being underpinned by multiple assumptions, only some of which are aligned to social justice and feminist principles.

Chapter 5 follows on from the critical analysis of the implications of the trauma concept, by presenting empirical interview data that further illustrates the contested meanings of trauma, and women's complex negotiations of medicalised and therapeutic constructions of gender-based violence. This chapter explores the ways in which therapeutic interventions provide a meaningful and yet flawed response to women's experiences of gendered oppression. Finally, Chapter 6 provides a number of suggestions for negotiating the contested trauma concept, including how notions of trauma within mental health settings can be harnessed to produce liberating outcomes for women. In addition, the chapter highlights the importance of finding opportunities for social action in response to gender-based violence, outside of the constraints of therapeutic and mental health service contexts.

References

American Psychiatric Association. (2013). *Diagnostic and statistical manual of mental disorders* (5th ed.). Arlington: American Psychiatric Publishing.

Anderson, S., Brownlie, J., & Given, L. (2009). Therapy culture? Attitudes towards emotional support in Britain. In A. Park, J. Curtice, K. Thomson, M. Phillips, & E. Clery (Eds.), *British social attitudes*. London: Sage.

Bateman, J., Henderson, C., & Kezelman, C. (2013). *Trauma-informed care and practice: Towards a cultural shift in policy reform across mental health and human services in Australia: A national strategic direction*. Retrieved from www.mhcc.org.au/media/32045/ticp_awg_position_paper__v_44_final___07_11_13.pdf.

Bath, H. (2008). The three pillars of trauma-informed care. *Reclaiming Children and Youth, 17*(3), 17–21.

Becker-Blease, K. A. (2017). As the world becomes trauma-informed, work to do. *Journal of Trauma & Dissociation, 18*(2), 131–138.

Bentall, R. P. (2010). *Doctoring the mind: Why psychiatric treatments fail*. London: Penguin Books.

Briere, J. N., & Scott, C. (2015). *Principles of trauma therapy: A guide to symptoms, evaluation, and treatment*. Los Angeles: Sage.

Burstow, B. (2018). 'Mental health' praxis not the answer – A constructive anti-psychiatry position. In B. M. Z. Cohen (Ed.), *Routledge international handbook of mental health* (pp. 31–38). London: Routledge.

Cleary, M., & Hungerford, C. (2015). Trauma-informed care and the research literature: How can the mental health nurse take the lead to support women who have survived sexual assault? *Issues in Mental Health Nursing, 36*(5), 370–378.

Crispin, J. (2017). *Why I am not a feminist: A feminist manifesto.* Brooklyn, NY: Melville House Publishing.

Foucault, M. (1980). *Power/knowledge.* New York: Harvester Wheatsheaf.

Fraser, N. (2009). Social justice in the age of identity politics. In G. Henderson & M. Waterstone (Eds.), *Geographic thought: A praxis perspective* (pp. 72–91). Abingdon: Routledge.

Gay, R. (2014). *Bad feminist: Essays.* New York: HarperCollins Publishers.

Gilfus, M. E. (1999). The price of the ticket: A survivor-centered appraisal of trauma theory. *Violence Against Women, 5*(11), 1238–1257.

Gnaulati, E. (2018). *Saving talk therapy: How health insurers, big pharma, and slanted science are ruining good mental health care.* Boston: Beacon Press.

Hooks, B. (2000). *Feminism is for everybody.* Cambridge: South End Press.

Josewski, V. (2017). A "third space" for doing social justice research. In M. Morrow & L. H. Malcoe (Eds.), *Critical inquiries for social justice in mental health* (pp. 60–86). Toronto: University of Toronto Press.

Kimmel, M. S. (2002). "Gender symmetry" in domestic violence: A substantive and methodological research review. *Violence against Women, 8*(11), 1332–1363.

Lacasse, J. R. (2014). After DSM-5: A critical mental health research agenda for the 21st century. *Research on Social Work Practice, 24*(1), 5–10.

Levenson, J. (2017). Trauma-informed social work practice. *Social Work, 62*(2), 105–113.

Lieggio, M. (2013). A denial of being: Psychiatrization as epistemic violence. In B. A. LeFrancois, R. J. Menzies, & G. Reaume (Eds.), *Mad matters: A critical reader in Canadian mad studies.* Toronto: Canadian Scholars Press.

Locke, T. (2004). *Critical discourse analysis.* London: Continuum International.

McLaughlin, H. (2008). What's in a name: 'Client', 'patient', 'customer', 'consumer', 'expert by experience', 'service user' – What's next? *The British Journal of Social Work, 39*(6), 1101–1117.

Moulding, N. (2015). *Gendered violence, abuse and mental health in everyday lives: Beyond trauma.* London: Routledge.

Moulding, N. T., Buchanan, F., & Wendt, S. (2015). Untangling self-blame and mother-blame in women's and children's perspective on maternal protectiveness in domestic violence: Implications for practice. *Child Abuse Review, 24*(4), 249–260.

Namy, S., Carlson, C., O'Hara, K., Nakuti, J., Bukuluki, P., Lwanyaaga, J., Namakula, S., Nanyunia, B., Wainberg, M. L., Naker, D., & Michau, L. (2017). Towards a feminist understanding of intersecting violence against women and children in the family. *Social Science & Medicine, 184*, 40–48.

North, C. E. (2006). More than words? Delving into the substantive meaning(s) of "social justice" in education. *Review of Educational Research, 76*(4), 507–535.

NSW Kids and Families. (2014). *Youth health resource kit: An essential guide for workers.* Sydney: NSW Kids and Families.

Poole, J. M., Jivra, T., Arslanian, A., Bellows, K., Chiasson, S., Hakimy, H., Pasini, J., & Reid, J. (2012). Sanism, "mental health" and social work/education: A review and call to action. *Intersectionalities: A Global Journal of Social Work Analysis, Research, Polity and Practice, 1*, 20–36.

Radford, J., Kelly, L., & Hester, M. (1996). Introduction. In J. Radford, L. Kelly, & M. Hester (Eds.), *Women, violence and male power* (pp. 1–16). Buckingham: Open University Press.

Reid, E. (2018). How the personal became political: The feminist movement of the 1970s. *Australian Feminist Studies, 33*(95), 9–30.

Rimke, H., & Brock, D. (2012). The culture of therapy: Psychocentrism in everyday life. In D. Brock, R. Raby, & M. P. Thomas (Eds.), *Power and everyday practices* (pp. 182–202). Toronto: Nelson Education.

Rose, N. (1998). *Inventing our selves: Psychology, power and personhood.* Cambridge: Cambridge University Press.

Rosenthal, M. N., Reinhardt, K. M., & Birrell, P. J. (2016). Guest editorial: Deconstructing disorder: An ordered reaction to a disordered environment. *Journal of Trauma & Dissociation, 17*(2), 131–137.

Sweeney, A., Clement, S., Filson, B., & Kennedy, A. (2016). Trauma-informed mental healthcare in the UK: What is it and how can we further its development? *Mental Health Review Journal, 21*(3), 174–192.

Taft, A., Hegarty, K., & Flood, M. (2001). Are men and women equally violent to intimate partners? *Australian and New Zealand Journal of Public Health, 25*(6), 498–500.

Thiara, R. K., & Gill, A. K. (2010). Understanding violence against South Asian women: What it means for practice. In R. K. Thiara & A. K. Gill (Eds.), *Violence against women in South Asian communities: Issues for policy and practice* (pp. 29–54). London: Jessica Kingsley Publishers.

Tseris, E. (2018). A feminist critique of trauma therapy. In B. M. Z. Cohen (Ed.), *Routledge international handbook of critical mental health* (pp. 251–257). Abingdon: Routledge.

Ussher, J. M. (2011). *The madness of women.* East Sussex: Routledge.

2 Interrogating biomedical dominance

Critical and feminist perspectives on mental health

In contemporary times, the identification of mental illness and the pursuit of mental health have become central preoccupations in the global north; meanwhile, the burgeoning agenda of "global mental health" has sought to increase the influence of psychiatric diagnostic practices and interventions on a worldwide scale. Despite the oft-repeated notion that mental illness is a hidden and under-recognised "silent epidemic", ideas about mental health difficulties currently infiltrate nearly every area of social life and are drawn upon to explain problems in an ever-expanding array of contexts, including at school, in workplaces, on the sporting field, in friendships, in family life, and in intimate relationships. Alongside the dual aims of maximising mental health and identifying "abnormal" mental states, the attempt to understand human experience on the level of genes and neurotransmitters is flourishing as both an area of academic research and, increasingly, within popular culture. Indeed, a biomedical viewpoint remains the most pervasive and influential explanatory framework of mental health, despite mounting evidence against the legitimacy of many of its claims, including serious concerns about "its adherence to reductionism, biological determinism, individualism, and unfounded notions of objectivity" (Malcoe & Morrow, 2017, p. 6).

As a response to intensifying debates and disquiet about psychiatric knowledge production, a range of alternative theories of mental health have emerged, offering avenues for exploring mental distress outside of biomedical hegemony. However, while many of these alternative theories of mental illness appear to value social explanations of distress, they are often limited by their ongoing acceptance of notions of individual "dysfunction", an insufficient analysis of how notions of mental health are shaped by power relations, and an over-reliance on therapy as a strategy for managing distress. Consequently, this chapter joins with other critical mental health scholars in advocating for the importance of *critical* mental health theorising, in order to provide a more comprehensive critique of both medical and therapeutic approaches to understanding distress (Cohen, 2018). Following this discussion, an overview of feminist perspectives on mental health and their role in highlighting the connections between psychiatric practices and gender inequality is provided. The discussions within this chapter set the scene for Chapter 3's more specific analysis of trauma-informed discourses in mental health settings, including how trauma discourses shape understandings of women's distress, and the extent to which the trauma paradigm has made a difference to women's empowerment and social justice outcomes in mental health settings.

Contested understandings of "mental illness"

Mainstream understandings of psychiatry situate the psychiatric profession as a medical specialty that is involved in the provision of high-quality treatment for individuals with mental disorders, based on rigorous scientific testing and assessment practices (American Psychiatric Association, 2014). Core assumptions underpinning the dominant biomedical model of mental illness include:

- mental illness is a substantial and rising problem, affecting increasing numbers of people every year;
- mental illnesses are brain-based diseases that are treatable primarily through medication, sometimes in combination with talking therapies, and;
- mental health assessments are based upon objective measurements of human behaviour and perceptions (Burstow, 2015; Wakefield, 2013).

In contrast to biomedical claims that position mental illness as a brain-based problem, critiques of biomedical psychiatry have examined the social contexts and professional practices that are important in explaining the rising numbers of people coming to the attention of mental health services. Such critiques have argued that increasing rates of mental health diagnosis reflect an ever-expanding Diagnostic and Statistical Manual of Mental Disorders (DSM), leading to an explosion in mental illness categories being used to describe experiences and behaviours that were previously accepted as part of the range of human experience (Gomery, Wong, Cohen, & Lacasse, 2011). Additions made to the most recent edition of the DSM that raised particular concerns include Disruptive Mood Dysregulation Disorder, referring to intense temper tantrums in children, Mild Neurocognitive Disorder, which arguably refers to "normal" ageing processes, and the removal of an exclusion criteria for Major Depressive Disorder in cases of recent bereavement, leading to arguments that grief has been medicalised in order to suit the agendas of pharmaceutical companies (Greenberg, 2013). Strikingly, the expansion of the DSM and the increasing influence of psychiatric knowledges has occurred in conjunction with a crisis of evidence facing psychiatry, and the failure to locate single biomarker for any mental disorder in the DSM (Deacon, 2013). Nevertheless, the numbers of people who are using psychiatric drugs continues to rise (Rose, 2016). The success of the biomedical discourse of mental health and its capacity to withstand such controversies can be traced in part to the aggressive marketing strategies of pharmaceutical companies that have influenced both the American Psychiatric Association (APA) and academic psychiatry (Whitaker & Cosgrove, 2015), with over two-thirds of the DSM-5 taskforce reporting ties to the pharmaceutical industry (Cosgrove & Krimsky, 2012). In addition, Moloney (2013) notes that increasing the number of diagnoses and reducing the threshold at which mental health interventions are offered serves the interests of mental health workers more broadly, as it expands the perceived scope of their professional expertise.

Nevertheless, the widespread influence of psychiatric discourses should not be viewed merely as resulting from the activities of pharmaceutical companies and professional bodies. Rather, the pervasiveness of psychiatric discourses is more comprehensively explained when considering the mutually beneficial relationship between the DSM and contemporary neoliberal political arrangements (Cohen, 2016). Neoliberalism can be defined as a political ideology based upon extolling the capacities of a free market to enhance human experience, leading to a diminishing of state responsibility for social welfare and a reformulated personhood premised on strong notions of individual responsibility, self-sufficiency, and enterprise – traits that enable people to become marketable assets (Sugarman, 2015). Sociological perspectives on mental health have noted the ways in which psychiatric practices converge with the power inequalities that are produced within neoliberal societies in a "brutal and destructive alliance" (Beresford, 2016, p. 343), by assessing and treating "dysfunctions" within individuals, rather than recognising the links between mental distress and social location, for example, the pivotal role played by experiences of poverty, violence, and discrimination in the development of mental distress. The solutions that are suggested by mental health discourses, such as medication and therapy to treat individuals, reflect neoliberal thinking, by transforming the distress caused by social risks including violence, child abuse, and poverty, into personal concerns (Kelly, 2010). In addition, traits including autonomy, emotional stability, sociability, and productivity are highly celebrated characteristics within neoliberal societies – as they are the traits of effective workers and consumers – and it is therefore little coincidence that mental health services are often aimed at developing these capacities, or intervening when these traits appear to be lacking (Esposito & Perez, 2014). Besides the successful lobbying of pharmaceutical corporations, then, the current dominance of the DSM can be traced to a neoliberal – and Eurocentric – preoccupation with productive and "rational" forms of personhood, and the capacity of the DSM to support neoliberalism by labelling as mentally unwell anyone who does not embody these attributes (Moncrieff, 2008). In this way, notions of "mental health", "wellbeing", and "mental illness" do not exist in a social vacuum, nor are they objective or timeless entities. Rather, they are informed by dominant social norms and power relations that elevate certain kinds of personhood above others (McLeod & Wright, 2016). Sugarman (2015) notes that the mental health professions have been slow to recognise their complicity with socio-political contexts, as it entirely undermines claims relating to the scientific neutrality of psychiatric knowledges.

Processes of disciplinary power are useful in understanding how some people may come to accept mental health labels as an appropriate explanation for their experiences, rendering their social worlds as invisible and irrelevant factors in understanding their mental distress. Foucault's work on disciplinary power notes that people in neoliberal societies do not merely absorb social norms and expectations; rather, they engage in active self-surveillance processes in an attempt to align to social norms and cultural ideals (Lafrance, 2007). According to Foucault (1980, p. 98):

> Power must be analysed as something which circulates . . . individuals circulate between its threads . . . they are not only its inert or consenting target; they are always also the elements of its articulation.

Thus, by identifying with and articulating dominant notions of mental health within their everyday lives, people extend the capacity of these discourses to explain their social and personal worlds (Gergen, 1999). As a result, psychiatric notions of "mental illness" act on people's lives and identities in complicated ways, by validating and legitimising experiences on the one hand (leading to access to mental health interventions and a straightforward explanation for their distress), as well as leading to potential disempowerment by providing only a narrow, individualistic view of complex social phenomena. Indeed, the dominance of psychiatric constructions is self-perpetuating, as service delivery is organised around diagnostic practices, contributing to their ongoing use in spite of hesitations that workers or service users may have about their suitability. This can lead to a sense that psychiatric notions are inevitable and that considering alternative approaches is unrealistic (Timmi, 2014). On the other hand, the relief felt upon receiving a diagnosis is frequently short-lived (British Psychological Society, 2011), and the resources opened up by a diagnosis may be overstated and are usually confined to medicalised or therapeutic support, rather than material resources or access to other forms of justice (Mills, 2015). In addition, although it would be misleading to suggest that mental health services are never useful, many people come to regret engaging with medical or therapeutic services due to their unhelpful, or even harmful effects (Ussher, 2018). Experiences of harm as a result of engaging with medical or therapeutic support continue to be alarmingly under-examined within mainstream mental health literature, and reflect a taken-for-granted assumption that access to mental health support is inherently beneficial.

Despite the emergence of a substantial critique of psychiatric practices – both within academic research contexts and more broadly – the dominant understanding of psychiatry remains, then, overwhelmingly a narrative of progress over time from ignorance to certainty and maltreatment to benevolence, with a strong belief in the efficacy of contemporary approaches in the form of pharmaceutical solutions, neuroscience imaging, and evidence-based therapies. Violent, bizarre, and misguided approaches to managing and responding to people named as mentally ill are seen as historical missteps, while contemporary practices including involuntary hospitalisation are viewed as necessary in order to manage "risky" individuals (Maylea, 2016). In contrast, mental health activists and critical theorists have persistently drawn into question comforting ideas about linear progress in mental health practice – without dogmatically denying evidence of progress, they have examined the ongoing harms that psychiatrised people continue to experience, exploring the connections between psychiatric practices and social inequalities, and interrogating the limitations of the claims made by contemporary psychiatric professionals, including objectivity and scientific rigour (LeFrancois, Menzies, & Reaume, 2013). The voices of mental health service users themselves have been a key element in the mounting of a persuasive critique of the limitations of psychiatric practices. Service users have challenged the systemic exclusion of their voices from mental health service provision, questioning the silences that have been created within mainstream psychiatric knowledge production (Brosnan, 2018). In contrast to a narrow biomedical focus on brain functioning, service user activism has emphasised the importance of experiential knowledges in opening up new perspectives on mental distress and difference, including an emphasis on social perspectives and the development of alternatives to involuntary treatment (O'Hagan, 2014). Service user activism has been pivotal in examining the ongoing limitations of contemporary mental health service provision, for example, the mixed consequences of de-institutionalised models of mental health service provision, which in many ways have replaced coercion with social neglect, through a dire lack of attention given to housing policies and welfare provision (Gooding, 2016). Furthermore, activists and critical mental health scholars have argued that Community Treatment Orders, as a substitute for involuntary mental health institutionalisation, merely replace one form of coercion with another, less visible form of social control:

> [P]eople can be restrained internally, through the body, as much as by external constraints or environmental barriers.
>
> (Fabris, 2016, p. 103)

There is, however, cause for some cautious optimism regarding the emergence of transformed understandings of "madness" and distress, outside of the dominant medical model. The World Health Organisation now recognises the need for a social analysis of mental distress, including the need to examine social inequalities rather than individual pathology:

> Levels of mental distress among communities need to be understood less in terms of individual pathology and more as a response to relative deprivation and social injustice, which erode the emotional, spiritual and intellectual resources essential to psychological wellbeing.
>
> (Freidli, 2009, p. iii)

In 2017, the United Nations called for major reform in mental health care, criticising diagnosing practices in relation to mental distress, questioning the conflation of mental distress with dangerousness, and challenging the notion that biomedical interventions are usually necessary (United Nations, 2017). Such sentiments reflect a growing disquiet with narrow biomedical viewpoint on mental distress, and an interest in broader explanations of distress located outside of a brain-based paradigm, including social, spiritual, and cultural explanations of mental distress and difference.

The questioning of an objective mental health lens has made way for alternative approaches to addressing mental illness that critique the dominance of biological perspectives in the mental health arena – perspectives that do not necessarily reject biological explanations, but interrogate the undue weight that has been given to them in comparison to other bodies of knowledge (Hall, 2016). For example, while critical psychiatrists do not deny the role of psychotropic medications in causing altered mental states, they have argued that they do not – as is commonly believed – act specifically to eliminate mental illness; rather, they cause general effects such as sedation (Moncrieff, Cohen, & Porter, 2013). Further, while neurobiological processes are involved in mental distress insofar as they enable people to experience emotional distress, this does not mean that biological processes *cause* distress (The Midlands Psychology Group, 2012).

Within the context of the biological sciences, feminist biologists have contended that while the "reality of nature" must be accepted to some extent, all ways of knowing about nature are at least partly socially constructed, as they are mediated by cultural and socio-political values and frameworks (Birke, 2000). In addition, Martin's (1991) anthropological work has shown the ways in which cultural tropes are routinely embedded within scientific accounts of biological processes, thus challenging the notion of neutrality within scientific knowledge processes. Issues relating to subjectivity and cultural biases are even more heightened in the mental health arena than in other contexts of biological investigation. For example, Johnstone et al. (2018) argue that the knowledge-gathering processes that are involved in psychiatric assessments are entirely different to those in the natural sciences, as they do not involve the measurement of objectively verifiable events and processes. Rather, mental health work is based upon developing "theories about the meanings of situations and actions . . . [therefore] the narratives constructed in therapy 'to an important extent . . . remain independent of facts'" (Spence in Johnstone et al., 2018, p. 83). This means that psychiatric practices involve highly ambiguous assessment processes, with workers' worldviews playing an integral part within mental health assessment processes (Burack-Weis, 2017). Nevertheless, the subjective nature of mental health practices, and their propensity to reflect and perpetuate dominant norms, including neoliberalism, remain peripheral within contemporary mental health literature.

Critical perspectives on mental health

Although social approaches to depression and anxiety are relatively well-known and somewhat accepted by mental health professionals and the broader community – especially if they are posited in conjunction with biomedical understandings – work has also begun on critiquing the dominant idea that the origins of experiences that are labelled as "psychosis" are entirely biological. For example, the International Society for Psychological and Social Approaches to Psychosis (ISPS) posits the need for a range of non-medical interventions in response to psychosis: "We believe that the preferred treatment of psychosis should be social and psychological interventions, with biological interventions (including medications) used sparingly" (ISPS, 2017, n.p.). Such statements are suggestive of an increasing interest in the development of more holistic approaches to understanding distress. Nevertheless, conceptualisations of mental illness that incorporate discussions about the social contexts of service users are frequently clustered together and viewed as an homogenous body of knowledge. The grouping together of diverse social theories can result in confusion, as social theories of mental health are not all in agreement about how mental distress should be understood or addressed. Examples include:

- Anti-stigma efforts, which often accept biological explanations and the legitimacy of psychiatric diagnoses, but argue for increased social acceptance and inclusion of people labelled as mentally ill (NoStigmas, 2017).
- Psychosocial approaches, which critique the effectiveness of psychotropic medication as a response to mental illness, exploring alternative responses, including self-help strategies, exercise, meditation, and so on (for example, Gordon, 2008).
- Social determinist arguments, which claim that mental illness is primarily caused by social inequalities, including poverty and social exclusion, rather than biological causes, thus attempting to explain the uneven patterns of mental illness diagnosis across society (Karban, 2017).
- Therapeutic approaches, which highlight the benefits of providing relational support to people through talking therapies, as an alternative to a medication response (Gnaulati, 2018).
- Neurodiversity arguments, based on the idea that people who have been labelled as mentally ill have differences (and different brains) that should be viewed as strengths, rather than illnesses or deficiencies (Armstrong, 2010).

Each of these positions has been useful in challenging the dominance of biomedical explanations of distress and developing more compassionate and less deficit-oriented responses to people labelled as mentally ill. However, critical perspectives on mental health take the evaluation of mental health discourses and practices further. Critical perspectives are necessarily broad and can be defined as "challenging the common sense, taken-for-granted view of what mental illness is . . . to problematise the mental health system, including the knowledge base and practices of mental health experts" (Cohen, 2018, p. 4). In contrast to the above approaches, which largely accept the legitimacy of the concept of mental illness, critical perspectives on mental health examine the ways in which the notion of mental illness is itself produced within particular social and political contexts, and is therefore open to contestation. This contrasts with anti-stigma campaigns, which usually attempt to increase mainstream diagnostic practices, by inviting people to understand themselves (and those around them) in terms of the language of mental health, for example:

It's easy and tempting to dismiss boredom as normal, especially given the stigma of mental illness.

(Komisar, 2018)

Anti-stigma campaigns that encourage people to seek help when distressed are premised on the assumption that the support that people receive will be useful, and by targeting "community attitudes" as the major impediment to quality of life for people diagnosed with mental illness, they neatly side-step the negative effects of psychiatric labels and interventions themselves. In contrast to the assertion that people in distress should seek professional help in order to become "well", critical perspectives acknowledge that sometimes the mental health assistance that people receive is unhelpful, or even harmful. While critical theories on mental health acknowledge that people who come to the attention of mental health services are often – though not always – experiencing serious distress, they are interested in examining the ways in which the diagnosing practices are "cultural tools used to understand different varieties of psychological distress and impairment" (Price-Robertson, 2018, n.p.), and they are interested in the uneven distribution of mental illness labels across society, wherein marginalised people (women, people of colour, people experiencing poverty, and so on) are more likely to receive a mental health diagnosis than people with more social power. Critical perspectives go further than considering how mental illness might be socially determined, however, by calling into question the very legitimacy of mental illness knowledge, and examining how mental illness diagnostic practices are involved in the mis-naming and re-interpreting of poverty, patriarchy, and racism in terms of individual dysfunction (Cohen, 2016). Such perspectives critique the ways in which social determinism, which still involves labelling individuals as mentally unwell, invites an individualising treatment response that ultimately shirks broader social change efforts:

[W]hile poverty may lead to psychological distress, correcting only the psychological issues will not necessarily correct the conditions of poverty that lead to the distress in the first place . . . it may actually allow such conditions to persist or worsen.

(Mills, 2015, p. 218)

Critical perspectives also extend neurodiversity arguments, which question the deficit-focus and lack of social analysis contained within mental illness diagnosing practices, but do not adequately challenge the practice of categorising people according to mental differences (Runswick-Cole, 2014). For example, neurodiversity arguments generally uphold the idea of the objective existence of mental differences – rather than situating the notion of mental differences as a social construction, bound by cultural values (Cutler, 2018). In addition, while critical mental health theories offer scathing critiques of the limitations of a diagnosis and medication response, they are also concerned about the limitations of therapeutic responses to mental distress, noting the ways in which therapeutic practices have the capacity to perpetuate neoliberal ideas in much the same way as a medicalised response. For example, therapeutic practices often continue to position individuals as dysfunctional, ignoring their social contexts, and failing to problematise the power relations between mental health professionals and service users:

> I soon discovered that it didn't matter whether biology or psychology won the battle for possession of my troubled mind. They were two sides of the same coin. Professionals who used either frame of reference were equally preoccupied with pathologizing my madness and with their futile attempts to get rid of it.
>
> (O'Hagan, 2014, p. 116)

Others have noted the ways in which the emphasis of therapeutic practices on individual behaviour change means that implicit within therapy is the assumption that individuals should accept and learn to manage social inequalities (Lee, 2017). In contrast, a fundamental component of critical mental health theory is an intersectional analysis, which is interested in the relationship between psychiatric oppression and other power relations, including racism, sexism, classism, heterosexism, and ableism (Wolframe, 2012). Such perspectives demonstrate that notions of "mental health" do not arise in a social vacuum, but are aligned with Eurocentric, masculine, and heterosexist norms and power relations, rendering marginalised groups as deficient:

> We are damaged by racism, by sexism, by classism, by hetersexism, by poverty and oppression. If our functioning is viewed in a vacuum, these factors are ignored, and we are seen as defective. If, instead, we are seen within the context of these factors, then efforts to help us will be much more meaningful and much less focused on our individual defects and pathologies. It makes little sense to ignore the society in which we all must live.
>
> (Chamberlin, 1995, p. 45)

As a result of this analysis, the notion of "global mental health" is positioned as a form of cultural imperialism, whereby Western notions of mental health are thought to be universally relevant and transferable across all cultural contexts (Summerfield, 2012). In contrast to a global mental health agenda, critical perspectives on mental health are interested in challenging the idea that notions of mental health are universally useful and transferable across contexts, and in highlighting the inadequacies of a Westernised model of mental health intervention that is premised upon changing the behaviours and perceptions of individuals.

The role of feminism in critiquing mainstream mental health

Feminist appraisals of psychiatry are a pivotal component of critical perspectives on mental health. The development of feminist critiques of mental health discourses is best viewed within the context of the broader women's liberation movement, having developed along a parallel course with feminist theories and activism. Feminist theory is valuable in challenging the de-contextualised nature of psychiatric knowledge about women's experiences:

> The gap between what I was learning in my classes at the university and the stories I heard from women at the other end of the crisis line about their experiences of violence disturbed and troubled me. So many of these women had stories about how they had been disbelieved by mental health professional when they had disclosed experiences of sexual and physical abuse. . . . Violence was not the only thing that marked many of these women's lives – poverty and experiences of racism and homophobia were also evident.
>
> (Morrow, 2007, p. 69)

Feminist mental health theorising is interested in both improving mental health practices through the rejection of patriarchal assumptions embedded within psychiatric discourses, as well as through the development of feminist mental health practices as an alternative to mainstream psychiatric practices (Enns, 2012). Such analyses have identified the ways in which psychiatric labels and treatments are not objective entities, but rather serve the function of social control. Feminist work in mental health has examined the multitude of mental health practices that have been involved in the problematisation of women and femininity, including but certainly not limited to Freud's pathologisation of female anatomy and his use of psychoanalytic concepts to reinforce patriarchal assumptions about the inferiority of women. In research settings, feminist theory has problematised the use of laboratory experiments and quantitative methods, and the absence of women's voices and experiences (Eagly & Riger, 2014). Chesler (1972, p. 116) argued that women who act out conditioned femininity are given psychiatric diagnoses such as depression, and that women who reject a conventional female role are nonetheless "assured of a psychiatric label" such as schizophrenia. Indeed, it has been long-recognised that definitions of mental health are aligned with stereotypically masculine traits and symptoms of mental illness often resemble stereotypically feminine traits (Broverman, Broverman, Clarkson, Rosenkrantz, & Vogel, 1981). Further, feminist critiques have highlighted the range of coercive mental health practices that have been developed as an attempt to control women's resistances to patriarchy (Ussher, 2011). By locating the cause of women's distress as an individual pathology, treatable through medical and therapeutic interventions, psychiatric practices are implicated in invisibilising social and political explanations of women's experiences.

In a contemporary context, the DSM contains "highly gendered psychiatric diagnoses such as postpartum depression, premenstrual dysphoric disorder, borderline personality disorder and female orgasmic disorder [which] serve to reinforce ascribed and socially accepted roles for women as obedient mothers, carers, workers and sexual partners" (Cohen, 2013, p. 12). Women outnumber men across a range of mood, sexual, personality, sleep, eating, adjustment, anxiety disorders, and post-traumatic stress disorder (PTSD) (Ussher, 2011). However, despite the mounting empirical evidence now available regarding the gendered dimensions of mental health diagnosing practices, mental health research continues to situate the causes of women's overrepresentation in the mental health system within biological or psychological dynamics. For example, feminists continue to contest the pathologising notion that women experience approximately twice the rates of depression and anxiety than men because they are biologically more vulnerable to mental illness, or because they have less "adaptive" coping mechanisms (Fullager & Gattuso, 2002; Taft, 2003). In contrast, feminist and social justice conceptualisations of women's overrepresentation within the mental health system have focused on examining the function of traditional sex roles that are imposed onto women within patriarchal societies, and the urgent need to attend to the sociopolitical contexts of women's emotional distress, which are obscured through diagnostic practices.

Third-wave feminism and psychiatry

The contributions of third-wave feminisms have introduced further nuances to a feminist analysis of psychiatric discourses and their effects on women. In addition to an analysis of gendered power relations, third-wave feminist theory is concerned with avoiding the totalising effects of rigid ideological positions, recognising diversity among women, and acknowledging women's resistances to oppression. Third-wave feminism has thus urged feminists to engage with complexities and nuances, while still finding ways to address questions about structural inequality (Phillips & Cree, 2014). Crucial to this work is a critique of the essentialism within earlier feminist perspectives, and a movement away from an all-encompassing notion of "womanhood", which reflects only the needs and perspectives of privileged, white, straight women and has historically excluded the voices of more marginalised women (Qin, 2004). In particular, women of colour, disabled women, and queer women have spoken strongly about the need for silenced perspectives within mainstream feminism to be interrogated, critiquing a meta-narrative about gender inequality that has resulted in an inability to explore "the intersecting forms of oppression that shape women's lives and multiple subject positions" (Razack in Thiara & Gill, 2010, p. 38). As a response to this critique, intersectional feminist theory has set out to reveal the partial and socio-historically situated production of second-wave feminist theory, to consider a range of other power relations in combination with gender, and to draw upon a diverse range of women's experiences and perspectives.

Also significant within third-wave feminism is the use of poststructural theory to reject neat certainties about women's experiences and to avoid deterministic explanations, whereby women are understood as wholly oppressed by patriarchal relations. A poststructural framework is interested in searching for multiple realities, based on the premise that "there are many ways to be a woman, and these ways are fluid, dynamic, and shaped by the intersectionality of categories of difference" (Quiros & Berger, 2014, p. 153). Rather than determining a new "truth" about women's experience, poststructural feminisms are interested in making space for multiple knowledges and understandings. In addition, a poststructural approach to feminism aims to identify not only how women are constituted by dominant discourses, but also the ways in which they actively engage with dominant discourses, both negotiating and resisting these discourses on an everyday basis. In this way, women's engagement with dominant discourses is framed as evidence of their strategic negotiation of power relations within highly constrained contexts, *not* as evidence that women have been deceived by patriarchal assumptions or that they have "internalised" patriarchal norms.

It has been noted that a poststructural approach to feminism may undermine the aims of feminist work, in that its focus on uncovering complexities and multiplicities seems misaligned with the aim of drawing attention to pervasive patterns of gendered inequalities and their effects. There have been concerns raised by some feminists that the use of poststructural theory will result in a loss of political power for women and that the feminist agenda of gender equality will become fragmented and ineffective, since within poststructuralism there can be no single understanding of terms such as *women* and there are considered to be multiple, diverse experiences of inequality. Indeed, Hanisch and Moulding (2011) note that poststructuralism has a "conservatizing" potential, whereby instead of adding complexity to second-wave feminism's descriptions of the harmful effects of gender-based violence, it can be used to completely undermine and de-politicise feminist claims about the intersections between gendered power and violence. This hazard is pertinent in relation to violence against women and children, given the multiple waves of backlash that have been directed towards feminist consciousness-raising efforts about the pervasiveness of gender-based violence (Herman, 1992). For example, since its emergence in the 1990s, the "false memory" movement's claims relating to the unreliability of adults' – in particular, women's – memories of child abuse, has enjoyed sustained interest despite being based upon exaggerated, misapplied and over-generalised research findings (Brewin & Andrews, in Salter, 2018). Moreover, men's rights activists have attempted to undermine policy agenda relating to women's safety and rights, based upon incorrect interpretations of statistical data that has resulted, for example, in the "gender symmetry" claim that family violence is perpetrated equally by men and women (Taft, Hegarty, & Flood, 2001).

Such concerns are particularly relevant in a contemporary era of "post-truth" politics (Khan & Wenman, 2017). Within such a context, it seems necessary to clarify that while poststructural analysis is interested in the processes through which particular forms of research come to be understood as representing the "gold standard" of evidence while other forms of evidence are de-legitimised, it does not view all claims to knowledge as holding equal weight (Graham, 2005), and it is deeply invested in exploring how knowledge claims are linked to practices of domination (Khan, 2017). Poststructuralism has been further critiqued for a "failure to deal with realities of the material world" (Feely, 2016, p. 866) – potentially focusing too heavily on strategies of deconstruction, identity politics or a "politics of recognition", at the expense of an embodied, structural analysis and re-distribution agenda (Josewski, 2017). Poststructuralism has emerged primarily within academic contexts that have historically suspended the body altogether (Fullagar & Pavlidis, 2018), prompting calls for a re-engagement with the embodied experiences of women as an intrinsic component of effective feminist activism alongside an analysis of discourses (Ussher, 2010). Additionally, the concerns of critical mental health theorists in how diagnostic practices both reflect and perpetuate societal power relations – for example, gendered, classed, and racialised inequalities – can be lost in some of the fragmenting and de-essentialising strategies within poststructuralism (Cohen, 2013).

Pulling together the contributions of multiple feminist perspectives involves harnessing the transformative and deconstructive potential of third-wave feminisms, while also finding ways to continue to meaningfully engage with women's distress and gendered power – "the ability to contest oppressive identity categories – whilst also exploring the actual material world . . . and the visceral experience" (Feely, 2016, p. 868). A key aim is to balance the generation of generalisable claims about social power, with the contributions of subjective lived experience knowledges (Josewski, 2017). In doing so, feminist theory retains its commitment to political action, while also being attuned to how political action can be co-opted by professional power, in order to create new therapeutic markets and diagnostic certainties. For example, a narrative about inevitable trauma following violence has been instrumental in developing community knowledge about the widespread problem of violence against women and children (Salter, 2018). However, the arguments offered within this book contend the trauma narrative has come at a cost, and work is now needed to revise its totalising tendencies. The trauma paradigm has led to the diverse and nuanced perspectives of women and children being invisibilised, while leaving dominant structures of medical and therapeutic power relatively intact, or in some cases, strengthened (Levett, 1992). Drawing on the work of Foucault, Alcoff and Gray (1993) note that while the act of "speaking out" has the capacity to transform power relations and subjectivities, it also necessitates that the narratives that people share are constructed within the constraints of dominant discourses, including medical and therapeutic expertise. This tension in activist work is key to an analysis of the emergence of the trauma paradigm in mental health in terms of its liberatory capacities for women, as well as concerns about its unintended exclusions and requirements – wherein women's narratives that do not neatly fit within the constraints of medical-therapeutic discourses risk being either silenced or diluted.

Concluding reflections

In contrast to a dominant view of mental illness, based upon notions of biological abnormalities, this chapter has reviewed a range of contestations in the mental health arena, with a particular focus on critical and feminist theories of mental health. Although many contemporary perspectives on mental health address the relevance of "social contexts" – for example, by discussing the need for stigma reduction, increased community awareness-raising and the adequate allocation of resources for research and frontline services, with some accounts even going so far as to examine the effects of the social world on the development of mental illness – a deeper analysis about the connections between mental health and social justice has remained relatively marginal. This chapter has explored the contributions of critical mental health perspectives in exploring how mental health discourses reflect and perpetuate dominant power relations including patriarchy, neoliberalism, and Eurocentrism. Further, it has argued that the concept of mental illness is not neutral, but is shaped by historical, cultural, and socio-political contexts and power relations.

The discussion in this chapter sets the scene for Chapter 3's exploration of the (re)emergence of trauma perspectives in mental health. Despite the burgeoning body of critical mental health scholarship that is asking essential questions about the political, social, and cultural contexts that underpin psychiatric knowledges, trauma-informed mental health practices have, to date, largely escaped the gaze of critical analysis. Indeed, trauma discourses have often been represented as the much-awaited antidote to the narrow vision offered by biomedical psychiatry. Trauma-informed mental health has been conceptualised as offering a *transformed* understanding of mental health service provision. Its current status in mental health settings is largely due to its role in replacing the idea that people in distress are affected by biochemical dysfunctions with the notion that people in distress have often endured unspeakable harms related to violence, oppression, or other devastating life events. Consequently, trauma-informed mental health approaches have been labelled as empowering, and – in relation to women's mental distress – politically progressive and aligned to a feminist perspective. Chapter 3 provides an in-depth investigation of these claims, arguing that while they have the capacity to embody these attributes, trauma-informed practices often continue to be constrained by the limitations of mainstream psychiatric assumptions and practices.

References

Alcoff, L., & Gray, L. (1993). Survivor discourse: Transgression or recuperation? *Signs: Journal of Women in Culture and Society, 18*(2), 260–290.

American Psychiatric Association. (2014). *About APA & psychiatry.* Retrieved from www.psychiatry.org/about-apa-psychiatry.

Armstrong, T. (2010). *Neurodiversity.* Cambridge: Da Capo Press.

Beresford, P. (2016). From psycho-politics to mad studies: Learning from the legacy of Peter Sedgwick. *Critical and Radical Social Work, 4*(3), 343–355.

Birke, L. (2000). Sitting on the fence: Biology, feminism and gender-bending environments. *Women's Studies International Forum, 23*(5), 587–599.

British Psychological Society. (2011). *Response to the American Psychiatric Association: DSM-5 development.* Retrieved from http://apps.bps.org.uk.

Brosnan, L. (2018). Who's talking about us without us? A survivor research interjection into an academic psychiatry debate on compulsory community treatment orders in Ireland. *Laws, 7*(4), 33–47.

Broverman, I. K., Broverman, D. M., Clarkson, F. E., Rosenkrantz, P. S., & Vogel, S. R. (1981). Sex-role stereotypes and clinical judgements of mental health. In E. Howell & M. Bayes (Eds.), *Women and mental health* (pp. 86–97). New York: Basic Books.

Burack-Weis, A. (2017). Introduction: Many ways of knowing. In A. Burack-Weis, L. S. Lawrence, & L. B. Mijanos (Eds.), *Narrative in social work practice: The power and possibility of story* (pp. 1–12). New York: Columbia University Press.

Burstow, B. (2015). *Psychiatry and the business of madness: An ethical and epistemological accounting.* New York: Palgrave Macmillan.

Chamberlin, J. (1995). Rehabilitating ourselves: The psychiatric survivor movement. *International Journal of Mental Health, 24*(1), 39–46.

Chesler, P. (1972). *Women and madness.* New York: Avon Books.

Cohen, B. M. Z. (2013). Psychiatric hegemony: A Marxist view on social constructionism. In F. Davies & L. Gonzalez (Eds.), *Madness, women and the power of art* (pp. 3–24). Oxford: Inter-Disciplinary Press.

Cohen, B. M. Z. (2016). *Psychiatric hegemony: A Marxist theory of mental illness.* London: Palgrave Macmillan.

Cohen, B. M. Z. (2018). Introduction: The importance of critical approaches to mental health and illness. In B. M. Z. Cohen (Ed.), *Routledge international handbook of critical mental health* (pp. 1–12). London: Routledge.

Cosgrove, L., & Krimsky, S. (2012). A comparison of DSM-IV and DSM-5 panel members' financial associations with industry: A pernicious problem persists. *PLoS Medicine, 9*(3), e1001190.

Cutler, E. (2018). *My complicated thoughts on neurodiversity.* Retrieved from www.radicalabolitionist.org/radical-abolitionist/2018/6/30/my-complicated-thoughts-on-neurodiversity.

Deacon, B. J. (2013). The biomedical model of mental disorder: A critical analysis of its validity, utility, and effects on psychotherapy research. *Clinical Psychology Review, 33*(7), 846–861.

Eagly, A. H., & Riger, S. (2014). Feminism and psychology: Critiques of methods and epistemology. *American Psychologist, 69*(7), 685–702.

Enns, C. Z. (2012). Feminist approaches to counseling. In E. M. Altmaier & J. C. Hansen (Eds.), *The Oxford handbook of counseling psychology* (pp. 434–459). Oxford: Oxford University Press.

Esposito, L., & Perez, F. M. (2014). Neoliberalism and the commodification of mental health. *Humanity and Society, 38*(4), 414–442.

Fabris, E. (2016). Community treatment orders: Once a rosy deinstitutional notion? In J. Russo & A. Sweeney (Eds.), *Searching for a rose garden: Challenging psychiatry, fostering mad studies* (pp. 96–108). Monmouth: PCCS Books.

Feely, M. (2016). Disability studies after the ontological turn: A return to the material world and material bodies without a return to essentialism. *Disability & Society, 31*(7), 863–883.

Foucault, M. (1980). *Power/knowledge.* New York: Harvester Wheatsheaf.

Freidli, L. (2009). *Mental health, resilience and inequalities.* Copenhagen: World Health Organisation.

Fullagar, S., & Pavlidis, A. (2018). Feminist theories after the poststructuralist turn. In *Feminisms in leisure studies* (pp. 48–71). London: Routledge.

Fullager, S., & Gattuso, S. (2002). Rethinking, gender, risk and depression in Australian mental health policy. *Australian E-journal for the Advancement of Mental Health, 1*(3), 2–13.

Gergen, K. J. (1999). *An invitation to social construction.* London: Sage.

Gnaulati, E. (2018). *Saving talk therapy: How health insurers, big pharma, and slanted science are ruining good mental health care.* Boston: Beacon Press.

Gomery, T., Wong, S. E., Cohen, D., & Lacasse, J. R. (2011). Clinical social work and the biomedical complex. *Journal of Sociology and Social Welfare, 38*(4), 135–165.

Gooding, P. (2016). From deinstitutionalisation to consumer empowerment: Mental health policy, neoliberal restructuring and the closure of the 'Big bins' in Victoria. *Health Sociology Review, 25*(1), 33–47.

Gordon, J. S. (2008). *Unstuck: Your guide to the seven-stage journey out of depression.* Australia: Hay House.

Graham, L. G. (2005). *Discourse analysis and the critical use of Foucault.* Paper presented at the Australian Association for Research in Education, Sydney.

Greenberg, G. (2013). *The book of woe: The DSM and the unmaking of psychiatry.* New York: Scribe Publications.

Hall, W. (2016). *Outside mental health: Voices and visions of madness.* United States: Madness Radio.

Hanisch, D., & Moulding, N. (2011). Power, gender and social work responses to child sexual abuse. *Affilia: Journal of Women and Social Work, 26*(3), 278–290.

Herman, J. L. (1992). *Trauma and recovery: The aftermath of violence – From domestic abuse to political terror.* New York: Basic Books.

ISPS. (2017). *ISPS Liverpool declaration.* Retrieved from www.isps.org/index.php/publications/isps-liverpool-declaration.

Johnstone, L., Boyle, M. with, Cromby, J., Dillon, J., Harper, D., Kinderman, P., Longden, E., Pilgrim, D. & Read, J. (2018). *The power threat meaning framework: Overview.* Leicester: British Psychological Society.

Josewski, V. (2017). A "third space" for doing social justice research. In M. Morrow & L. H. Malcoe (Eds.), *Critical inquiries for social justice in mental health* (pp. 60–86). Toronto: University of Toronto Press.

Karban, K. (2017). Developing a health inequalities approach for mental health social work. *British Journal of Social Work, 47*(3), 885–992.

Kelly, P. (2010). Youth at risk: Processes of individualisation and responsibilisation in the risk society. *Discourse Studies in the Cultural Politics of Education, 22*(1), 23–33.

Khan, G. (2017). Beyond the ontological turn: Affirming the relative autonomy of politics. *Political Studies Review, 15*(4), 551–563.

Khan, G., & Wenman, M. (2017). The politics of poststructuralism today. *Political Studies Review, 15*(4), 513–515.

Komisar, E. (2018). *Don't dismiss a new mum's boredom. It could be a sign of something more serious.* Retrieved from www.smh.com.au/lifestyle/life-and-relationships/don-t-dismiss-a-new-mum-s-boredom-it-could-be-a-sign-of-something-more-serious-20180731-p4zumu.html.

Lafrance, M. N. (2007). A bitter pill: A discursive analysis of women's medicalized accounts of depression. *Journal of Health Psychology, 12*(1), 127–140.

Lee, D. A. (2017). A person-centred political critique of current discourses in post-traumatic stress disorder and post-traumatic growth. *Psychotherapy and Politics International, 15*(2), e1411.

LeFrancois, B. A., Menzies, R. J., & Reaume, G. (Eds.). (2013). *Mad matters: A critical reader in Canadian mad studies.* Toronto: Canadian Scholars' Press Inc.

Levett, A. (1992). Regimes of truth. *Agenda, 8*(12), 67–74.

Malcoe, L. H., & Morrow, M. (2017). Introduction: Science, social (in)justice, and mental health. In M. Morrow & L. H. Malcoe (Eds.), *Critical inquiries for social justice in mental health* (pp. 3–30). Toronto: University of Toronto Press.

Martin, E. (1991). The egg and the sperm: How science has constructed a romance based on stereotypical male-female roles. *Signs, 16*(3), 485–501.

Maylea, C. (2016). An end to involuntary treatment in Australian mental health social work. In N. Paul & P. Jones (Eds.), *Social work and health: Inclusive practice research and education* (pp. 94–119). Kerala: Depaul Centre for Research and Development.

McLeod, J., & Wright, K. (2016). What does wellbeing do? An approach to defamiliarize keywords in youth studies. *Journal of Youth Studies, 19*(6), 776–792.

Mills, C. (2015). The psychiatrization of poverty: Rethinking the mental health – Poverty nexus. *Social and Personality Psychology Compass, 9*(5), 213–222.

Moloney, P. (2013). *The therapy industry: The irresistible rise of the talking cure, and why it doesn't work.* London: Pluto Press.

Moncrieff, J. (2008). Neoliberalism and biopsychiatry: A marriage of convenience. In C. I. Cohen & S. Timini (Eds.), *Liberatory psychiatry: Philosophy, politics and mental health* (pp. 235–256). New York: Cambridge University Press.

Moncrieff, J., Cohen, D., & Porter, S. (2013). The psychoactive effects of psychiatric medication: The elephant in the room. *Journal of Psychoactive Drugs, 45*(5), 409–415.

Morrow, M. (2007). Critiquing the "psychiatric paradigm" revisited: Reflections on feminist interventions in mental health. *Resources for Feminist Research, 32*(1/2), 69–85.

NoStigmas. (2017). *The NoStigmas project.* Retrieved from https://nostigmas.org/nostigmas-project/.

O'Hagan, M. (2014). *Madness made me.* Wellington: Open Box.

Phillips, R., & Cree, V. E. (2014). What does the 'fourth wave' mean for teaching feminism in twenty-first century social work? *Social Work Education, 33*(7), 930–943.

Price-Robertson, R. (2018). *Diagnosis in child mental health: Exploring the benefits, risks, and alternatives.* Retrieved from https://aifs.gov.au/cfca/publications/diagnosis-child-mental-health.

Qin, D. (2004). Toward a critical feminist perspective of culture and self. *Feminism and Psychology, 14*(2), 297–312.

Quiros, L., & Berger, R. (2014). Responding to the sociopolitical complexity of trauma: An integration of theory and practice. *Journal of Loss and Trauma, 20*(2), 149–159.

Rose, N. (2016). Neuroscience and the future for mental health? *Epidemiology and Psychiatric Sciences, 25*(2), 95–100.

Runswick-Cole, K. (2014). 'Us' and 'them': The limits and possibilities of a 'politics of neurodiversity' in neoliberal times. *Disability & Society, 29*(7), 1117–1129.

Salter, M. (2018). Finding a new narrative: Meaningful responses to 'false memory' disinformation. In V. Sinason (Ed.), *Memory in dispute.* London: Karnac.

Sugarman, J. (2015). Neoliberalism and psychological ethics. *Journal of Theoretical and Philosophical Psychology, 35*(2), 103–116.

Summerfield, D. (2012). Afterword: Against "global mental health". *Transcultural Psychiatry, 49*(3–4), 519–530.

Taft, A. (2003). *Promoting women's mental health: The challenges of intimate partner/domestic violence* (Issues Paper 8). Australian Domestic and Family Violence Clearinghouse. Retrieved from www.austdvclearinghouse.unsw.edu.au/PDF%20files/Issues_Paper_8.pdf.

Taft, A., Hegarty, K., & Flood, M. (2001). Are men and women equally violent to intimate partners? *Australian and New Zealand Journal of Public Health, 25*(6), 498–500.

The Midlands Psychology Group. (2012). Draft manifesto for a social materialist psychology of distress. *Journal of Critical Psychology, Counselling and Psychotherapy, 12*(2), 93–107.

Thiara, R. K., & Gill, A. K. (2010). Understanding violence against South Asian women: What it means for practice. In R. K. Thiara & A. K. Gill (Eds.), *Violence against women in South Asian communities: Issues for policy and practice* (pp. 29–54). London: Jessica Kingsley Publishers.

Timmi, S. (2014). No more psychiatric labels: Why formal psychiatric diagnostic systems should be abolished. *International Journal of Clinical and Health Psychology, 14*(3), 208–215.

United Nations. (2017). *World needs "revolution" in mental health care – UN rights expert.* Retrieved from www.ohchr.org/EN/NewsEvents/Pages/DisplayNews.aspx?NewsID=21689.

Ussher, J. M. (2010). Are we medicalizing women's misery? A critical review of women's higher rates of reported depression. *Feminism & Psychology, 20*(1), 9–35.

Ussher, J. M. (2011). *The madness of women.* East Sussex: Routledge.

Ussher, J. M. (2018). A critical feminist analysis of madness: Pathologising femininity through psychiatric discourse. In B. M. Z. Cohen (Ed.), *Routledge international handbook of critical mental health* (pp. 72–78). London: Routledge.

Wakefield, J. C. (2013). DSM-5 and clinical social work: Mental disorder and psychological justice as goals of clinical intervention. *Clinical Social Work Journal, 41*, 131–138.

Whitaker, R., & Cosgrove, L. (2015). *Psychiatry under the influence.* New York: Palgrave Macmillan.

Wolframe, P. M. (2012). The madwoman in the academy, or, revealing the invisible straightjacket: Theorizing and teaching saneism and sane privilege. *Disability Studies Quarterly, 33*(1).

3 The mainstreaming of trauma in mental health

Radical critique, or business as usual?

The previous chapter explored the benefits of applying feminist and critical mental health theories to mental health settings in order to explore the limitations of psychiatric discourses in explaining mental distress. By drawing into question notions of psychiatric objectivity, it investigated the involvement of psychiatric discourses in both reflecting and perpetuating social oppressions, including gender inequality. In addition, it explored a diverse array of alternative conceptualisations of mental health that have attempted to extend the narrow perspective offered by psychiatry. This present chapter turns its attention specifically to trauma-informed practices in mental health, which are widely thought to provide more holistic and empowering understandings of mental health service users in comparison to mainstream psychiatric practices. The aim of this chapter is to evaluate the extent to which such claims about trauma-informed practices in mental health are being realised, particularly in relation to women presenting to mental health services with experiences of gender-based violence. This chapter draws upon and extends a small body of literature that has advocated for heightened caution relating to the proliferation of the trauma concept in mental health.

The discussion in this chapter converges with my own shifting engagement with the trauma paradigm, which commenced as a largely complacent adoption of trauma-informed ideas as a social worker engaging with young women diagnosed with mental health difficulties. This initial acceptance has transformed into a present-day apprehension about the burgeoning use of trauma as an organising narrative for conceptualising women's suffering. I am now convinced that there is an urgent need to think critically about the constraints of the trauma paradigm as a way of understanding and responding to mental distress. While my initial reactions to the notion of trauma in mental health settings were characterised by a hopeful enthusiasm for its potential alignment to feminist values and its capacity to critique biomedically saturated mental health systems, this has been followed by a persistent unease about the hazards and limitations involved in using trauma to enact emancipatory outcomes for women.

My engagement with trauma discourses commenced during a time of employment in a child and adolescent mental health service, where I was experiencing the agency's emphasis on diagnosis, risk assessment, symptom checklists, and medication of children and young people jarring to my social work training. My studies in social work had emphasised some of the principles of critical and feminist theories that were discussed in the previous chapter, including the need for an analysis of power in addition to (or as a replacement for) diagnostic processes, and I was committed to the idea of taking the experiences of service users into account when considering the origins of their distress and what could be done about it. The disjuncture inspired me to delve into alternative, socially oriented approaches to understanding the difficulties that I saw service users facing. In particular, I was concerned about the ways in which young women who were engaging in self-harming behaviours attracted the frustration of mental health workers, in part because their "symptoms" often appeared to be much more intractable in comparison to more "straightforward" presentations, and also because frequently these young women did not want to attend the service, but were referred by their parents or teachers. As a result, they were unwilling and sometimes uncooperative recipients of mental health support and they did not always express gratitude for the assistance that was being offered. Consequently, they represented a dangerous and irritating mix of "risky" behaviours and "non-compliance". Labels, medications, treatment plans, and risk checklists would ensue – responses that provoked a rising disquiet in me and led me on a search for a different approach.

It did not take me long to come across the work of trauma researchers including Judith Herman (1992) and John Briere (1992), who offered sharp analyses of the effects of early-life events, especially the effects of ongoing exposure to violence and abuse, on the lives of people who come to the attention of mental health services. Herman's (1992) work outlined the lack of attention given by mainstream psychiatric services to the effects of exposure to abuse and violence. Instead of a reliance on pathologising and de-contextualised psychiatric labels, Herman proposed a new diagnostic category, complex post-traumatic stress disorder (C-PTSD), which aimed to situate service users' symptomotology within a context of prolonged exposure to adverse events of an interpersonal nature. Although post-traumatic stress disorder (PTSD) examines the effects of external stressors, Herman argued that it did not adequately account for the complexities of repeated experiences of violation, for example, the long-term implications of childhood victimisation. Additionally, Briere and his colleagues discussed the effects of childhood maltreatment on adolescent and adult psychological functioning, making links between experiences of abuse and symptoms such as self-harm and suicidality (J. Briere & Jordan, 2009; J. Briere & Lanktree, 2012). In response, I began to conceptualise my work with young women who had been labelled with depression, anxiety and personality disorders through a trauma lens. The trauma paradigm assisted me to understand the meanings behind service users' "symptoms", giving me the confidence to re-classify their experiences as "immense sadness", "fear and terror", and "extreme distress" in response to overwhelming situations of abuse, and the related experiences of shame and powerlessness. Indeed, this points towards one of the most important aspirations of trauma-informed mental health – the aim to shift the focus from service users' intrapsychic worlds and to consider their social contexts when attempting to sense the distress that they are experiencing (R. D. Goodman, 2014).

Despite the seeming escape from the medical model that was offered by the trauma concept, and the meaningful conversations that occurred when sharing these ideas with the young women I was working with, I began to think also of the harm that could be caused by holding onto the alternative "trauma-informed" explanatory narrative too strongly. David Smail's provocative book *How to Survive without Psychotherapy* (1996) argues that in many instances, mental health workers gain more benefits from service users than service users from them. Indeed, it was in my conversations with the young women who I was charged to "help" that I first discovered the need to critique the assumptions underpinning my new-found commitment to trauma discourses, and to ask questions including:

- What am I to make of the experiences of a significant proportion of the young women who I am meeting, which defy categorisation – with even Herman's notion of complex post-traumatic stress disorder being too deficit-oriented and prescriptive in its scope?
- What am I to do when young women tell me that they do not think that they are "traumatised"? If I continue to insist that they are, just how different is the trauma discourse to any other kind of diagnostic labelling practice?
- Where is the space within trauma work to talk of the young women's courage, and their fierce determination to live meaningful, flourishing adult lives? What about their humour, intelligence, and compassion, in spite of what they have experienced?

It was at this point that I started to critically engage with the category of the "traumatised" woman, including some of its embedded assumptions and values. Stepping back from the immediacy of practice, it becomes apparent that the use of "welfare words" locate problems inside individuals and cultivate comforting and yet unrealistic certainties around complex human experiences (Garrett, 2018). Although the "traumatised" label provided some acknowledgement of gender-based violence as a serious social problem – a welcome reprieve from the historical denial and minimisation of its impacts – I noticed that it could also be oppressive, regardless of its intentions. Through developing a template for capturing women's psychological responses to abuse, it mimicked conventional diagnostic practices in mental health of "fixing" service users into rigid categories. Over time, my interactions with service users convinced me that the trauma discourse is, as Gavey and Schmidt term, "a double-edged template", which is "potentially othering, stigmatizing, [and] violating" (2011, p. 433). Young women had their own ways of talking about their experiences, and I was humbled by their hope-filled plans for the future, combined with their resolute critique of taken-for-granted ideas about the social world (*Why are things this way, and how could things be organised more fairly?*) Interestingly, such social critique is often constructed as overly idealistic, and evidence of an immature "stage" of development on the pathway to adult ways of being, including a more accepting perspective (Frankel, 1998). I began to notice how a preoccupation with confining young women's experiences to the narrow parameters offered by trauma theory often undid their own meaning-making processes and resulted in the effects of violence being seen as linear, prescriptive, and absolute. The complex implications of the trauma paradigm in mental health contexts form the focus of this chapter's analysis.

The (re)emergence of trauma

Notions of trauma, and trauma-informed practices, are frequently understood as markedly new concepts within contemporary mental health service provision, and yet the assertion of "newness" within the human services should be interrogated as a suspicious epistemological claim (Butler in Zhang, 2017). Indeed, trauma theory has a history dating at least as far back as the late nineteenth century in early psychoanalytic theory. Prior to his abandonment of seduction theory, Freud understood "hysterical" symptoms in women to be the result of the psychic trauma caused by childhood sexual abuse, which he wrote about in *The Aetiology of Hysteria* (Taft, 2003). Hypnosis was used as a strategy to access and transform these traumatic memories (Haaken, 1998). However, following the criticism he received in response to this work – in particular, the incredulity that such large numbers of women could have experiences of sexual assault – Freud revised his theory that hysteria was caused by sexual abuse, instead theorising that women's memories of childhood sexual assault were fantasies (Masson, 2012). From this point onwards, Freud took on the prevailing patriarchal views of his period, arguing that women are anatomically, psychologically, and morally deficient compared to men, with underdeveloped superegos, and he abandoned his investigation into trauma (Brandell, 2004). Freud's turnaround would come to have a sustained, damaging influence on mental health practices relating to women, contributing to the ongoing invisibilisation of women's experiences within psychiatric contexts, and a de-contextualised analysis of their distress (Taft, 2003). Several decades would pass before the trauma concept was thoroughly re-examined within psychiatric literature.

The effects of the First and Second World Wars prompted a resurgence of interest in trauma theory in the twentieth century – for men, this time, rather than women – due to emerging evidence of the long-term psychological distress experienced by returning soldiers (Courtois, 2004). The trauma concept aimed to create a language and a method for understanding the effects of exposure to war, including nightmares and flashbacks, which previously had not been named or properly understood (Humphreys & Joseph, 2004). The turn towards trauma signalled a significant paradigm shift: mental distress was viewed not only as a problem for a small, deficient proportion of the population, but a condition that could be experienced by anyone, given exposure to significant stress (Scull, 2011). In contrast to previous constructions of "shell shock" that had emphasised psychic weaknesses and pre-disposing factors within affected soldiers, PTSD repositioned distress in war veterans as primarily arising from exposure to warfare, a shift in understanding that has become so well-accepted that warfare is now widely thought to be inextricably linked to the development of mental distress (Roberts-Pedersen, 2015).

Post-traumatic Stress Disorder (PTSD) was first included in the third edition of the *Diagnostic and Statistical Manual of Mental Disorders*, published in 1980. Once the PTSD diagnosis was available, it began to be strategically used by feminist therapists to describe issues relevant to women's mental health. However, feminists expressed concerns about the notion contained within the DSM-III that PTSD arises from an event beyond the range of normal human experience, arguing that gender-based violence is in fact a common experience affecting large proportions of girls and women (Brown, 1991). This specification was removed from subsequent editions of the DSM. In the DSM-5, a person can be diagnosed with PTSD if they have been exposed to death, threatened death, actual or threatened serious injury, or actual or threatened sexual violence, including through indirect exposure, such as in the course of professional duties (American Psychiatric Association, 2013). In determining a diagnosis of PTSD, the DSM specifies that a person be experiencing functional impairments or distress for more than one month, related to:

- reexperiencing (for example, through nightmares or flashbacks);
- avoidance of trauma-related thoughts, feelings, or reminders;
- negative thoughts or feelings, which began or worsened after the event;
- arousal and reactivity that began or worsened after the event (for example, hypervigilance or difficulty sleeping).

As mentioned in Chapter 1, a distinction is often – though not always – made between trauma resulting from isolated, non-interpersonal events, and *complex* trauma resulting from long-term experiences of violence or abuse, of a relational nature (including child abuse, neglect, and gender-based violence), often involving experiences of betrayal (Rosenthal, Reinhardt, & Birrell, 2016). Developmental Trauma is an alternative term in use to describe the effects of violence, abuse or neglect in early childhood. However, despite significant advocacy relating to the inclusion of separate complex or developmental trauma diagnoses in addition to PTSD, such a diagnosis was not added into the DSM-5 – although Complex PTSD is included in addition to PTSD in the World Health Organisation's *International Statistical Classification of Diseases and Related Health Problems*, 11th Edition (ICD-11). Changes that were made to PTSD in the DSM-5 include the location of PTSD in a new category of disorders, *Trauma and Stressor Related Disorders*, alongside Reactive Attachment Disorder, Disinhibited Social Engagement Disorder, Acute Stress Disorder, and Adjustment Disorder – a shift from its previous classification as an Anxiety Disorder.

The ongoing exclusion of complex and developmental trauma from the DSM has been condemned by researchers and workers who claim that the PTSD diagnosis is severely limited in its capacity to conceptualise experiences such as rape and abuse (van der Kolk, 2017). In particular, there have been concerns raised about the inability of the PTSD symptom list to adequately capture the effects of long-term, interpersonal violence (Herman, 1992). Such concerns reflect the widespread notion that psychiatric diagnoses are useful in legitimising distress and potentially enabling service users to access the resources that they need.

However, the attempt to expand the DSM to include yet another diagnostic category sits uncomfortably within a critical mental health paradigm that is concerned about the already excessive capacity of the DSM to construct human experiences as abnormal. An engagement with the DSM in order to develop mental health services that are able to more fully capture the needs of women may preclude a more comprehensive critique of psychiatric practices and an exploration of non-psychiatric responses to gender-based violence. As the trauma concept is largely enacted from within the constraints of mainstream mental health services, there are hazards involved in its attempt to provide de-pathologising and emancipatory outcomes. Several limitations of trauma discourses and their implications for women are addressed in the second half of this chapter. Prior to this, the core principles of the trauma paradigm are outlined in more detail, followed by an analysis of some of the hopeful aspects of the increasing proliferation of trauma-informed practices in contemporary mental health settings.

Core principles of trauma work

Judith Herman's seminal text, *Trauma and Recovery* (1992) outlined three stages of response to complex trauma: safety and stabilisation; remembrance and mourning; and reconnection and integration. Several authors have modified and expanded upon Herman's model of trauma, and there is now a proliferation of trauma therapies that have been developed as specific interventions to assess and alleviate the "symptoms" of trauma. In a model based on "current, continuous, and cumulative" trauma, Kira, Ashby, Omidy, and Lewandowski (2015) outline eight principles: prioritising safety; addressing threats through behaviour skills training; stimulating the will to live and positive dispositional qualities; identity work; psychoeducation; stress inoculation; trauma narration; and advocacy, social justice and reconnecting to social networks. The National Child Traumatic Stress Network (nd) outlines a number of steps for conducting an assessment of complex trauma, including: assess for a wide range of traumatic events; assess for a wide range of symptoms, risk behaviours, functional impairments, and developmental derailments; and try to make sense of how each traumatic event might have impacted developmental tasks and derailed future development. Trauma-informed care was developed out of an aim to create human service settings that could be helpful and respectful for service users with histories of violence and other overwhelming experiences, which they may not disclose. It comes from an awareness that a majority of mental health service users have experienced violence, abuse or other overwhelming stressors at some point in their lives, and that mental health services can cause further harm through coercive and disempowering practices (Muskett, 2014). Trauma-informed principles include aspirations relating to safety, trust, collaboration, choice, and empowerment (Levenson, 2017). In an expanded model, Elliott, Bjelajac, Fallot, Markoff, and Reed (2005) outline ten principles of trauma-informed services:

- recognise the impact of violence and victimisation on development and coping strategies;

- identify recovery from trauma as a primary goal;
- employ an empowerment model;
- strive to maximise service users' choice and control;
- strive for relational collaboration with survivors;
- create an atmosphere that is respectful of survivors' need for safety, respect, and acceptance;
- emphasise service users' strengths, highlighting adaption over symptoms;
- minimise the possibilities of re-traumatisation through avoiding invasive questioning;
- strive to be culturally competent;
- solicit service user input in designing and evaluating services.

It is difficult for anyone who is frustrated by the reductionism within mainstream psychiatric service provision to not be initially excited by the possibilities entailed within contemporary trauma discourses and their refreshing re-conceptualisation of the tenets of biomedical psychiatry. In particular, the trauma paradigm is credited with shifting the emphasis within mental health services away from the question, "what is wrong with you?" to the alternative question, "what has happened to you?" (Longden, Madill, & Waterman, 2012).

Nevertheless, in naming trauma-informed practices as a "new" paradigm of mental health care, their resemblance to the psychodynamic paradigm has been significantly understated. Trauma-informed practices mirror a psychodynamic approach in a number of important ways: most notably, they mirror the psychodynamic idea that rather than viewing disturbances in thoughts and behaviours as arising merely from an unwell brain, mental health workers should explore service users' experiences in detail, in order to unravel important clues about the origins of their distress (Scull, 2011). Nevertheless, the contemporary trauma paradigm can be differentiated from a psychodynamic approach in two major ways: it draws heavily on biological discourses, including brain imaging, as a way of providing evidence for its efficacy; and it emerged within a context of feminist activism relating to the treatment of women within mental health services and beyond, including concerns about the unrecognised prevalence of gender-based violence and its effects. The major claims made by trauma-informed approaches are discussed in more detail below, allowing for an exploration, firstly of how the trauma concept has made way for more empowering responses to women, and secondly, the ongoing limitations of the trauma paradigm relating to the realisation of women's rights within mental health services.

Transformed perspectives on violence and women's experiences

Notwithstanding a raft of evidence that has repeatedly contradicted the connection, a spurious link between mental illness and violence is an entrenched and long-standing cultural trope, which has led to a raft of both microaggressions and systemic discriminatory practices against people labelled with a psychiatric diagnosis. The link between mental illness and violence has remained intact despite evidence demonstrating the much higher likelihood that mental health service users have been victims rather than perpetrators of violence (Bentall, 2010). Although the unfounded association is often framed as being located within the imaginations of an "uneducated" lay community, mental health professionals themselves are in fact deeply involved in perpetuating a risk, violence, and mental illness nexus. For example, mental health legislation is premised upon an understanding that people diagnosed with mental illnesses pose excessive risks to themselves and others, while people without a mental illness diagnosis who engage in behaviours that could easily be constructed as "risky" are more likely to escape this level of surveillance and regulation; furthermore, mental health discourses are invested in sustaining the construction of psychiatric dangerousness in order to justify involuntary treatment (Maylea, 2016). People with racialised identities are further oppressed by this construction, as counter-terrorism strategies attempt to connect notions of "psychological vulnerability" with the risk of radicalisation (Coppock & McGovern, 2014).

A preoccupation with assessing for the risk posed by individuals with mental health diagnoses has, for a long time, acted as a distraction from the systemic violence that is perpetrated within mental health systems themselves, in the form of hospitalisation, seclusion, and restraint, as well as a variety of other coercive practices enacted within both voluntary and involuntary settings (Clarke, Barnes, & Ross, 2018; Ross, 2018). Such practices have largely escaped scrutiny, due to a taken-for-granted assumption about the "presumed prudence" of mental health professionals (van Daalen-Smith, Adam, Breggin, & LeFrançois, 2014). Considering the gendered dimensions of psychiatric harm specifically, Burstow frames electroconvulsive therapy (ECT) – an intervention that is applied at vastly disproportionate rates to women – as a form of violence against women due to the impairments that it causes and the function that it performs in silencing women's stories of abuse (Burstow, 2006). Psychiatry is further implicated in violence against mental health service users due to its role in ignoring the link between distress and social oppressions. In place of a social analysis, mental health assessments frequently involve only de-contextualised symptom analysis and an assessment of the risks posed by individual service users' mental states and behaviours.

The trauma concept has obvious uses in countering these limited perspectives, through providing an overdue acknowledgement of the violence that has been experienced by a large proportion of mental health service users, which has historically remained undetected within mental health assessments (Trevillion, Corker, Capron, & Oram, 2016). This acknowledgement has led, in some instances, to changed practices in psychiatric settings, including enhanced screening of service users for past and present experiences of violence, including sexual assault, child abuse, and other adverse events (Cusack, Frueh, & Brady, 2004). Rather than merely representing a risk to self or others due to their diagnoses, the trauma concept re-positions service users as potentially at risk of harm from others, allowing for their distress to be seen within its broader social context, and for referrals to be made to services offering practical supports rather than merely mental health interventions. In addition, the trauma paradigm has revealed the propensity of mental health workers to use strategies that reflect or exacerbate the abuse that service users have experienced, for example, the use of an authoritarian style or problem-focused assessment processes (NSW Kids and Families, 2014). Trauma-informed service provision calls for the development of collaborative partnerships between service users and professionals, a strengths-based approach, and a reduced use of psychiatric labels in favour of more contextualised understandings of mental distress. The use of the trauma concept to understand women's mental health concerns is often positioned as intrinsically connected to social justice, through its recognition that service users are affected not merely by internal biological processes, but also by their life histories and social environments (Knight, 2015). These changed practices aim to reduce the risk of service users experiencing further trauma ("re-traumatisation") as a result of mental health interventions. Although somewhat basic, such changes challenge long-standing practices of coercion within mental health services, which have often been invisibilised through assumptions about the benevolence of the mental health professions.

Trauma and respecting women's experiences

Through its different approach to understanding and responding to distress, the trauma paradigm has the capacity to counteract a range of humiliating practices inflicted upon women within psychiatric contexts. Borderline personality disorder (BPD) is widely understood to be one of the least useful and most disparaging mental illness labels in the DSM, where it is defined as "a pervasive pattern of instability of interpersonal relationships, self-image, and affects and a marked impulsivity beginning by early adulthood and present in a variety of contexts", with the symptom list including frantic attempts to avoid abandonment, unstable and intense interpersonal relationships, unstable sense of self, impulsivity, recurrent suicidal behaviour or self-harm, affective instability, chronic feelings of emptiness, difficulty controlling anger, paranoid ideation, and dissociation (American Psychiatric Association, 2013). BPD is, without doubt, a gendered psychiatric diagnosis, with women receiving a BPD diagnosis much more frequently than men, with the ratio being as high as 9:1 (Eriksen & Kress, 2004). Its symptomatology reflects stereotypically feminine traits including emotionality, relational dependence, instability, irrationality, and unreliability, reflecting Ussher's (2013) assertion that constructions of femininity are intrinsically connected to constructions of madness. There is also a patent subjectivity involved in the assessment of BPD. For example, how exactly is an "intense" interpersonal relationship defined? What constitutes a "frantic" effort to avoid abandonment, as opposed to an "ordinary" or "normal" effort? Why is it that women are branded with the BPD diagnosis, when stalking, threats and intimidation, and violence following relationship separation are acts that are overwhelmingly perpetrated by men towards women?

As discussed in Chapter 2, questions have been raised about the effectiveness of psychiatric medications for a vast range of mental illness diagnoses, however the ineffectiveness of psychoactive drugs in alleviating any of the "symptoms" associated with BPD is especially apparent (Lieb, Völlm, Rücker, Timmer, & Stoffers, 2010). The significant prejudices that women with the BPD diagnosis have been subjected to within the mental health system have been well-documented. People with BPD report being castigated when seeking support from the mental health system and advised that they are using resources that rightly belong to people with legitimate health concerns (Latalova, Ociskova, Prasko, Sedlackova, & Kamaradova, 2015). The inability of a mainstream medical model to make a difference to women's presentations goes some way to explaining the construction of women with BPD as manipulative and undeserving service users, who are "not really mentally ill" (even though the brains of women diagnosed with BPD have been a topic of scientific research). The self-harm and suicidal behaviours of women with BPD are frequently constructed by mental health workers as "attention-seeking" behaviours rather than as a sign of serious emotional distress. As noted by Kulkarni (2015, n.p.):

> The word "borderline" was used in the 1930s by psychoanalysts to describe patients whose symptoms were on the border between psychosis and neurosis. But today the most common interpretation of the word is that the condition "borders" on being a real illness.

Consequently, once diagnosed as mentally unwell, the reality and severity of distress experienced by women with a BPD diagnosis continues to be called into question. Thus, women with a diagnosis of BPD are situated in a position of double oppression: they experience all of the damaging effects of psychiatric labelling, without any of the potential benefits that a mental health diagnosis can incur, in terms of social validation or sympathy. It has been suggested that women may be more frequently diagnosed with BPD due to a bias in diagnosing practices, whereby mental health workers are more likely to consider environmental factors affecting men's distress, while understanding women's distress as caused by their internal states (Becker & Lamb quoted in Eriksen & Kress, 2004). Adding further to this context of gendered oppression, the diagnosis of BPD has been shown to be strongly connected to experiences of chronic child abuse (Wagner & Linehan, 1994), a context that is entirely invisibilised within DSM language. As a result of this strong correlation, the BPD diagnosis has been condemned for participating in the concealment of women's survival strategies and social protest in relation to gender-based violence, by re-naming their resistance as mental illness (Nicki, 2016). This practice mirrors the processes involved in Freud's abandonment of his investigations into sexual assault in favour of describing women's accounts of sexual violence as mere fantasies.

Therefore, feminist appraisals of psychiatric practices have been scathing in their critiques of psychiatry's collusion with patriarchal power, and psychiatry's facilitation of the silencing of women's dissent against gendered oppression. On first glance, the trauma concept appears to offer a vastly improved conceptualisation of women's distress, wherein women's voices are privileged, their accounts are believed, the significance of gender-based violence in shaping mental distress is validated, and mental health services aim to offer collaborative and non-judgemental support. PTSD is one of the few diagnoses in the DSM that discusses the role of social context in the emergence of distress. As a result of an awareness about trauma-informed mental health, medical professionals are implored to consider the relevance of gender-based violence in women's mental health presentations (Rees & Fisher, 2016). Both the diagnosis of PTSD and the broader trauma paradigm in mental health settings have opened up increased spaces for previously ignored feminist approaches, including a commitment to elevating women's strengths rather than the deficit-focus of mental illness diagnostic frameworks; breaking down power imbalances and providing non-coercive responses wherever possible; evaluating patterns of social power rather than individual experiences of distress in isolation; and refuting the notion that the disproportionate numbers of women who become mental health service users is evidence of biological vulnerabilities or merely women's high propensity for "help-seeking" behaviours. Mental health workers are no longer able to dismiss women's distress if they have been labelled with a BPD diagnosis on the basis that they appear to lack a strong basis in biology, as trauma provides a coherent social explanation. In fact, the trauma paradigm may mean that the pejorative BPD diagnosis is drawn upon much less frequently, with "complex trauma" being preferred as a more compassionate and accurate descriptor for women's experiences in the aftermath of violence.

Trauma beyond the DSM: intergenerational and collective trauma

In contrast to other psychiatric labels, notions of PTSD and complex PTSD give much-needed attention to the social contexts of mental distress, with the capacity to shift the focus of mainstream mental health practices from internal dysfunctions to external stressors. However, their ongoing role in identifying symptoms in individuals results in a restricted scope for examining the social relations of power that are important in making sense of patterns of violence and structural inequalities. In response to these limitations, efforts have been made to expand the trauma concept beyond the parameters of the DSM, to include attention to ecosystemic and socio-political factors, as well as how the trauma concept can be used in ways that are relevant across diverse socio-cultural contexts (R. Goodman, 2013). Contrasting with the DSM's attempt to identify mental pathologies, notions of collective, historical, and intergenerational trauma critique the individualistic focus of psychiatric diagnoses, instead considering the structural contexts of violence (Oudshoorn, 2015). For example, the concept of intergenerational or transgenerational trauma has been used by Indigenous scholars to describe the ongoing effects of dispossession, with a focus not only on harm, but also on processes of survival, courage, and hope (Atkinson, 2002). This application of the trauma concept has provided a powerful counterpoint to the devastating ways in which mental health discourses have pathologised Indigenous people and communities, making space for an interrogation of the ways in which psychiatric discourses distil the vast and ongoing effects of structural racism to the level of individual "symptoms". In this way, trauma-informed practices have enabled a strong critique of the overrepresentation of Indigenous people as mental health service users, and the role played by psychiatric labels in mis-naming the effects of violence, genocide, and racism. In addition, the trauma paradigm's role in elevating Indigenous worldviews, knowledge, and cultural strategies has been instrumental in addressing the tendency for mental health services and policies to exclude the perspectives of Indigenous people (Josewski, 2017).

At the same time, Linklater's (2014) discussion of decolonising trauma work emphasises the ongoing limitations of trauma discourses in attaining social justice outcomes, given that the term "trauma" originates from Western contexts; furthermore, trauma implies personal rather than state responsibility, and despite attempts for a more expansive trauma discourse, discussions relating to trauma for the most part continue to centre on the DSM and diagnoses such as PTSD. This analysis is important in examining a number of concerns that have been raised by critical mental health scholars about the limitations of trauma-informed discourses in mental health. For example, Caplan (2016) critiques the default responses of diagnosis, therapy and medication that are provided to people who are understood to be experiencing trauma:

> Why should it be considered a mental illness to be devastated by war, assault, or other traumatic experiences? And if that is a mental illness, then what would be a mentally *healthy* response be to death, moral horror, or major life losses?

Continuing this line of analysis, the next section of this chapter details a number of hesitations that have been raised by critical scholars about the implications of trauma discourses for women who have experienced gender-based violence. This discussion considers the effects on women of the increasing utilisation of the trauma concept in mental health services, providing a critical appraisal of the extent to which the trauma paradigm has resulted in a shift towards the enactment of feminist and social justice values and practices.

Symptoms and essentialising constructions

Since the (re)emergence of the trauma concept within mental health settings, the "trauma" experienced by women as a result of violence has been extensively researched. The psychological problems that have been connected to repeated and prolonged exposure to gender-based violence are thought to extend well beyond the PTSD symptoms of reexperiencing, experiential avoidance and hyperarousal, to include difficulties with chronic affect dysregulation, self-harming behaviours, substance abuse, dissociative problems, problems in relating to others and "boundary" issues between self and others, irritability, somatisation, and distortions in concepts about self and others – a symptom list that "can be prolonged almost indefinitely" (Herman, 1992, p. 123). The research agenda into trauma symptomatology, which emphasises pathologies and dysfunctions within survivors of abuse and violence, seems to be at odds with widespread claims made about the "empowering" or de-pathologising capacities of trauma-informed practices. Implicit within much of this research is an assumption that exposure to events that are labelled as traumatic will lead, in a predictable fashion, to psychological problems, which is evident in van der Kolk's (2017, p. 401) assertion that:

> [C]hildren exposed to alcoholic parents or domestic violence rarely have secure childhoods; their symptomatology tends to be pervasive and multi-faceted and is likely to include depression, various medical illnesses, and a variety of impulsive and self-destructive behaviors . . . a vast system of internal disorganization.

The strong link between violence and trauma is now well-entrenched within both social and professional understandings. It was enormously important to feminist activism during the twentieth century in countering notions about the non-harmful nature of violence against women and children, and this advocacy was especially urgent in the area of child sexual assault. However, while the violence-trauma nexus has produced useful benefits by enabling women's experiences of distress to be validated, it has also led to deterministic and essentialising notions about women possessing definite and irreversible vulnerabilities after trauma (Haaken, 1998). The notion of universal trauma effects is informed not only by psychiatric discourses, but also by essentialising assumptions within some feminist theorising that has not engaged well with the diversity of women's experiences (Gavey & Schmidt, 2011). Nevertheless, it is the symptom orientation of mental health services that has been fundamental in the development of a narrow view on the effects of violence, and a disappearing social analysis:

> [W]hile there was initially a level of exchange between feminism and the helping professions on the subject of gendered violence and its effects, the direction of this has become increasingly one-directional with many feminist practitioners now drawing on psychological concepts such as "trauma" but arguably few mainstream practitioners drawing on feminist understandings of gendered violence and abuse.
>
> (Moulding, 2015, p. 7)

Feminist scholars have noted the many deleterious consequences of the emphasis on women's vulnerabilities after violence, including the assumption that women are helpless as a result of their trauma, leading to paternalistic practices, in ways that mimic mainstream psychiatric labelling practices. Commenting on the very early stages of the proliferation of trauma-informed practices, Debi Brock (1991, p. 14) astutely predicted, "women who reveal themselves to have been sexually abused when young risk having this become constructed as the crux of their identity – considered the formative experience of who they are".

It has been noted that Herman's (1992) portrayal of women survivors of violence developing a pattern of intense and unstable relationships in later life is also implicated in invoking a highly deterministic and pathologising view of abused women, whose social and relational skills are positioned as severely lacking (Todd, Wade, & Renoux, 2004). This analysis has entered into popular accounts of traumatised women, who are purported to "seek out" abusive men within their future relationships. Within this view, it is the survivor's damaged personality traits, distorted beliefs, and behaviours that lead her to be "re-victimised" in later life, rather than the prevalence of gender-based violence within society. While a critique of the "unstable" trauma survivor within Herman's work is warranted, given that Herman's analysis does at times lean heavily on symptom assessment, *Trauma and Recovery* explicitly asserts the need for trauma work to occur within the context of a social movement to end patriarchy. It is worthwhile to note how little regard this key argument in her book is given, in comparison to the sections on diagnosis and symptoms.

Alongside this deviation from Herman's politicised approach to trauma is evidence of another departure, within some trauma-informed practices, from the key principle of safety. There is now a broad consensus within the literature on trauma that mental health services should ask service users about their experiences to violence and abuse, among other experiences that are understood to be "traumatic". As described earlier in this chapter, the importance of safety is embedded within most iterations of trauma-informed mental health practices. In line with this principle, disclosure by service users to human service professionals has been described as a process, wherein service users are provided with choices relating to how, when, and to whom they make a disclosure of violence (NSW Kids and Families, 2014). Sweeney, Clement, Filson, and Kennedy (2016) discuss the need for skilled work in managing service users' disclosure of violence or other traumatic events, arguing that workers must be careful to move at the pace of service users, to give forewarning about trauma questions, and to allow service users the space not to answer them. As the trauma concept has become more mainstream, however, a different approach has emerged relating to the need for universal trauma screening practices that are more prescriptive in their approach, proposing the need to utilise checklists and validated screening tools to allow for "proper identification" that occurs "early in treatment" (Center for Substance Abuse Treatment, 2014). The introduction of trauma screening and assessment tools, as well as treatment protocols to be followed after a disclosure, can be viewed in part as an attempt to increase the visibility and perceived importance of violence and its effects within mental health service provision. Nevertheless, the tools draw heavily on the language of a mainstream biomedical approach and are explicitly concerned with the goals of the reliable identification of trauma symptomatology, accurate diagnosis, and treatment planning (see Kretschmar, Butcher, Tossone, & Beale, 2016). Questionnaires are designed to be "quickly administered", for example, the Brief Trauma Questionnaire (BTQ):

> asks respondents for a simple "yes" or "no" answer to the question "Have you experienced this event?" and lists ten types of traumatic events. For each "yes" response, the respondent is also asked two additional "yes/no"

questions: "Did you think your life was in danger or you might be seriously injured?" and "were you seriously injured?" The BTQ is designed to quickly screen for many different and prevalent types of traumatic experiences, including war traumas, serious car accidents, natural disasters, exposure to violent death, life-threatening illness, and physical or sexual abuse.

(Behavioral Health Evolution, 2016, n.p.)

Rather than reducing a reliance on notions of mental disorder in favour of descriptive and meaningful narratives, the identification of trauma is linked to "trauma-related symptoms and disorders" that must be "detected early and treated effectively" (Center for Substance Abuse Treatment, 2014). In these examples, while the notion of trauma exerts some influence on how the causation of mental distress is being understood and managed, it does so in a way that ultimately fails to disturb the everyday assumptions and practices of mental health service provision. Trauma practices based within an assessment and treatment paradigm seem to involve an astounding departure from some of the core principles of the trauma paradigm relating to safety, choices, and sharing power between workers and service users, instead reinstating the importance of the therapeutic "expert" who utilises a directive and hierarchical approach. Within these conceptualisations, there is a distancing from Herman's notions of empowerment:

The first principle of recovery is empowerment of the survivor. She must be the author and arbiter of her own recovery. Others may offer advice, support, assistance, affection, and care, but not cure. Many benevolent and well-intentioned attempts to assist the survivor founder because this basic principle of empowerment is not observed.

(Herman, 1992, p. 133)

The focus on symptoms and the development of a linear trajectory between violence and trauma can be further problematised by examining how it has led to the development of new hierarchies of distress and exclusions in mental health contexts. For example, trauma discourses have tended to focus on re-conceptualising only a narrow range of mental health diagnoses, while largely ignoring others, with feminist mental health workers rightly showing how depression, anxiety and personality disorders are mental health labels that are frequently imposed upon women who are simply expressing the distress caused by patriarchal oppression. Meanwhile, much less attention has been given to the possible connections between other kinds of "mental illness" experiences, such as hearing voices, and gender-based violence. Instead, such experiences have been understood as "serious" or "real" mental illnesses, in comparison to trauma reactions (Hunter, 2018). This demarcation is problematic: it ignores evidence relating to the effects of adverse life experiences on the development of a range of reactions, including what is generally labelled as psychosis (Longden & Read, 2016); and it de-pathologises some mental disorders, while strengthening the perceived validity and biological basis for others (Hanisch & Moulding, 2011). In addition, as the trauma discourse measures the veracity and seriousness of violence by its effects, women whose experiences in the aftermath of violence deviate from a picture of straightforward harm or trauma reactions face the risk of their experiences of oppression being met with disbelief (Smith & Woodiwiss, 2016). In other instances, the violence-trauma link may mean that women who have not faced gendered interpersonal violence but who have nonetheless faced gendered oppressions in other less obvious forms risk having their experiences of patriarchal violence go unnoticed or dismissed. As noted by an anonymous service user (2018, p. 14), "I'm unconvinced that all service users will identify a life defining trauma or be able to answer the proposed question, 'What happened to you?' methodically". This means that the trauma concept may place women with less clear-cut experiences of gendered oppression at risk of having their distress understood as biological, innate, or without a meaningful social context. Thus, despite the usefulness of the trauma paradigm in shifting some understandings of service users' experiences, women who are unable to articulate a linear trajectory between violence and mental distress may face ongoing difficulties in being heard and barriers to receiving compassionate mental health responses. Consequently, I cautiously concur with the argument that it is necessary "to broaden and deepen understandings of the whole spectrum of traumatic and adversarial life experiences that can lead to the development of extreme forms of distress" (Dillon, Johnstone, & Longden, 2014, p. 227). However in taking this more comprehensive view, there is a need for the diverse power relations and socio-political contexts underpinning the range of events that can be labelled as "traumatic" to be adequately differentiated from one another. The de-politicising tendencies of an overly broad and genericised view on trauma are outlined further in Chapter 4.

Trauma subjectivities, therapy, and neoliberalism

As described in Chapter 2, neoliberalism can be defined as an ideology that views an unregulated economy as the ideal means for enhancing social life, leading to a shrinking welfare state, and the championing of notions of individual responsibility, consumerism, productivity, and profitability (Esposito & Perez, 2014). While mainstream psychiatric practices support a neoliberal agenda, the trauma paradigm seems to offer a counter-narrative, by highlighting the socio-political contexts of women's lives, critiquing the de-contextualised and dehumanising effects of psychiatric labels, and inviting women to disclose their previously silenced stories of abuse and violence. The shift from silencing women's voices to making space for women's lived experiences has been linked to outcomes of empowerment and justice. For example, some writers have noted the resources and solace offered within "therapeutic cultures" where therapy is common, and where the techniques of therapy (including self-disclosure and open communication) are promoted outside of formal therapy settings as important life skills for managing difficult circumstances (McLeod & Wright, 2009; Swan, 2008). Thus, therapeutic and story-telling practices provide a form of social support for suffering that might otherwise be managed in isolation (Wright, 2008).

In contrast to this optimistic reading, there are connections between trauma-tised subjectivities and the neoliberal strategy of reducing structural inequalities to the level of individual minds. For example, Yasmin Nair (in Kinnucan, 2014) argues that a person who identifies as traumatised is an ideal neoliberal subject, because while personal narrative-making about trauma takes on the appearance of political critique, it reduces an analysis of systemic oppressions to a personal confessional practice. This means that when women speak about their experi-ences of gendered abuse either within therapy or in a more public context, it is not necessarily the case that feminist goals relating to empowerment and a structural analysis of power will automatically follow. Instead, an emphasis is placed on individual survivors, at the expense of perpetrators and – even more importantly – at the expense of a recognition of the political and cultural forces that support rape and gendered violence to continue (Hengehold, 2000).

As also outlined in Chapter 2, mental health discourses support neoliberal values through privileging the responsibilisation of individuals. The pressure to access therapy after adverse life events in order to manage emotional distress – a pressure which is heightened when other kinds of resources or forms of support are unavailable – is reflective of a strong moral imperative towards managing problems through individual efforts (Moloney, 2016). Thus, although they may be experienced as supportive, therapeutic discourses are also involved in placing expectations on women to take control of the "self" in order to be less emotional, more autonomous, more productive, and to overcome the effects of social inequal-ities (Brunila, 2014). Such pre-determined therapeutic goals reduce the capacity for therapeutic practices to engage with women's dissent in relation to patriarchal power relations. Critical perspectives on therapy have argued that despite prom-ises about the empowering capacities of the therapeutic relationship, therapy is actually highly limited in its capacity to promote women's liberation, due to its focus on personal change and adaptation to inequality, rather than consciousness-raising or social activism (McLellan, 1995).

Naples (2003) uses the term "recovery industry" to describe the cultural shift that has been occurring from the late twentieth century, wherein complete societal silence surrounding child abuse is transformed into the development of public and "uncensored" revelations of child abuse both within popular media and public contexts beyond therapy. In a similar vein, Armstrong (1994, p. 3) argues that therapy may use "noise to achieve the same end that was once served by repres-sion", creating isolated stories of "ventilation", due to a failure to adequately con-textualise the experiences or to address issues of power and injustice. In other words, experiences of abuse are spoken of, but women's narratives are positioned as personal tragedies that are not situated within a broader context of gender ine-quality. Fernandes (2016) argues that the contemporary turn towards story-telling practices can invite complacency, through the assumption that merely making space for narratives is sufficient to enact social justice outcomes. Narratives that are disconnected from their broader socio-political contexts may in fact fall well short of an aim of invoking radical social change, instead leading to passive empa-thy (Boler, 1997). The minute details of the abuse that are discussed may result in women being left with a sense of overwhelming isolation and vulnerability, in the absence of a validating social response (Gavey & Schmidt, 2011). Further, story-telling practices may result in women facing new forms of precarity, as women experience pressure to share publicly from their lived experiences in order for their perspectives on gender inequality to be heard, which may in turn lead to their analysis being taken less seriously (Razer, 2016). Mental health activists have argued that the replacement of silencing practices with compulsion to disclose personal experiences is simply another form of oppression:

> We believe being made to feel like you have to tell your "story" to justify your experience is a form of disempowerment, under the guise of empowerment.
>
> (Recovery in the Bin, n.d., n.p.)

The connection between the trauma paradigm and neoliberalism is even clearer when the trauma concept is merely used in conjunction with conventional mental health practices, rather than as a broad critique of the assumptions underpinning mainstream medicalised and therapeutic responses to women's distress. In a welcome shift from pathologising mental health language, the trauma paradigm sometimes – though certainly not always – chooses to replace the notion of "symptoms" with a construction of women's distress as not merely evidence of biologically based dysfunctions, but as "coping strategies" and "understandable reactions" to overwhelming stressors. Nevertheless, trauma practices often continue to position women as in need of professional treatment to resolve their reactions, which are understood to be no longer adaptive or relevant once abusive experiences have ended. Such conceptualisations presume that once women are no longer facing immediate danger, any residual safety concerns and distress that they may hold are evidence of "dysfunctional", or "maladaptive" beliefs. Burstow (2003), however, rails against the notion of "maladaptive" trauma responses that are in need of therapeutic repair, whereby a woman's lack of trust, ongoing concerns about safety, and beliefs relating to unfairness are considered to require a therapeutic intervention, rather than representing a realistic understanding of the dangers faced by women who may no longer have contact with a perpetrator of violence, but who nonetheless face ongoing risks within victim-blaming and patriarchal societies. More generic models of trauma-informed services on first glance appear to side-step the pathologisation of service users, by focusing on organisational changes towards trauma-sensitive services, rather than individual treatment. However, such approaches are still involved in positioning "traumatised" service users as problematic – they are understood as requiring an environment that is adequately "containing" in relation to any problematic trauma reaction that may emerge (Becker-Blease, 2017). In this way, women who express anger or distress within trauma-informed services risk having their views dismissed on the basis that they are experiencing a trauma reaction. Despite the aspirations and espoused values of the trauma-informed practices, such responses seem perilously similar to the difficulties faced by women with personality disorder diagnoses in having their distress met with compassion or their views taken seriously.

In contrast to the individualising effects of the trauma paradigm, and therapeutic practices more broadly, a range of critical and politicised approaches to therapy have attempted to develop radical re-conceptualisations of mainstream mental health services that privilege a socio-political analysis – while at the same time accepting that a large proportion of human service responses occur on a one-to-one level. For example, feminist therapies have been specifically constructed in response to the pathologising effects of both medical and conventional therapeutic practices, with the aim of positioning therapy as a potential site for consciousness-raising and the enactment of political action, allowing for women's so-called "symptoms" to be understood as resistance to patriarchy, and privileging feminine ways of relating to disrupt notions of the therapist-as-expert (Burstow, 1992). In a similar way, narrative therapy explicitly situates mental distress as related to external power relations rather than internal dysfunctions, allowing service users to develop understandings of the "self" outside of the language of deficit and pathology (White, 1995). Response-based practices have also disrupted normative mental health practices by highlighting the difference made by a positive *social* response to disclosures of violence, and interrogating the role of language in concealing violence against women, blaming survivors, and decreasing survivors' dignity by obscuring their resistances (Wade, 2014).

Within these critical approaches to mental health service provision, the gap between socio-political activism and therapy is not completely resolved, but is narrowed. Burstow (1992), however, warns of the tendency for some feminist therapists to hold onto psychiatric concepts that have oppressive implications for women, for example, accepting and using the language of diagnostic categorisation, or drawing upon therapeutic modalities without examining their inconsistency with feminism. In addition, a crucial question arising from politicised approaches to therapy is how to acknowledge the helpful aspects of individual identity work, while also working towards more substantial mental health reform and the broader goal of transforming social relations of power (Bottrell, 2009). Therapeutic responses – even at their most radical – enacted in the absence of broader political work risk shifting the onus of responsibility onto individuals alone to cope within inherently unbearable social conditions. On the other side of this argument is the claim that "feminist therapists create revolution insidiously, one person at a time" (Hill, 1998, p. vii), through making space for radical conversations within the constraints of mental health services that offer very limited – if any – support for group work and community practices, let alone a macro-level approach to activism. Similarly, Johnson (2012) cautions against reductionist socio-political critiques that offer only *explanations* for distress, or macro-level routes to addressing despair. Therefore, the role and scope of politicised therapeutic practices in addressing gender inequality and empowering women who have experienced patriarchal oppression and violence remains a contested area.

Trauma and constructions of resilience

In contrast to an essentialising narrative about trauma symptomatology, there exist more nuanced analyses of the effects of violence that do not view traumatic reactions as inevitable, but rather as a function of an enormous range of variables including stressor characteristics such as unpredictability and duration, alongside victim-survivor characteristics such as age, family context, socio-economic status, and previous experiences (J. N. Briere & Scott, 2015). Others have argued that while "traumatic events" are incredibly common – affecting the majority of people at some point in their lifecourse – PTSD emerges in only a minority of people (Friedman, 2015). Contrasting with a psychiatric deficit-orientation, some scholars have documented the various, often hidden ways in which women resist and respond to gendered oppression, offering a counter-narrative to the portrayal of dysfunction following violence (Wade, 1997). In addition, research documenting the possibilities of resilience, recovery, and even post-traumatic growth following violence and other adverse events is becoming increasingly common (Joseph & Linley, 2008). Upon first glance, this optimistic literature appears to offer much more empowering constructions of violence and trauma outside of the symptom preoccupation and deficit-focus offered by psychiatric discourses.

In a contemporary context, notions of recovery and resilience are now routinely included within mental health policy documents and practice guidelines, often but not always in combination with trauma discourses. Importantly, however, the recovery movement in mental health did not originate from within mainstream services, but was initially formulated in the mid-twentieth century from the perspectives of service users (Ahern & Fisher, 2001). This activism denounced the pervasive hopelessness embedded within mainstream psychiatric service provision, calling for a drastically transformed service system and the radical notion of peer-led support conducted outside the bounds of formal mental health programmes (O'Hagan, 2014). Worryingly, mental health activists have argued that the insertion of the "recovery" concept into contemporary service provision often represents an appropriation of the original concept rather than a genuine attempt to transform the power relations in mainstream mental health services. Mental health activists have argued that the apparently transformative turn in mental health settings from notions of lifelong illness to a focus on the possibilities of recovery and resilience is an example of an activist concept being subsumed into mainstream mental health discourses, and utilised for conservative purposes (Harper & Speed, 2012). In many cases, recovery has become a prescriptive imperative for service users to aspire towards, leading to new forms of oppression in spite of the history of the concept (Pilgrim & McCranie, 2013). Service users are expected to engage in the dual tasks of following the advice of mental health experts, while also exercising their own individual responsibility, in order to strive towards the achievement of recovery; meanwhile, the social and gendered dimensions of distress are ignored (O'Brien, 2012). Indeed, scant attention has been given to the socio-political conditions that may impede the possibility of recovery from distress within mainstream resilience research (Ungar, 2011). In this way, notions of recovery or resilience after violence should not be seen as an unproblematic means of empowering women and countering psychiatry hegemony.

The contested nature of recovery leads to questions relating to who should decide when someone has recovered, with service users, mental health workers, and family members likely to define recovery in different ways (Wallcraft & Hopper, 2015).

Further, the ill-defined bounds of recovery means that it is a concept that is open to wide interpretation – while it is possible for recovery discourses to act as a means of women's emancipation outside of a symptom-focus, notions of recovery can also be defined as the ability to manage without support (Roy, Rivest, & Moreau, 2016). As a result, recovery discourses are implicated in placing expectations on women to find ways to cope within contexts of unbearable, ongoing social inequalities (Bottrell, 2009). In addition, ideas about what counts as resilient behaviour, growth or strengths are not neutral, but are deeply embedded in dominant power relations and the norms and values of neoliberal societies. As noted by Rose (in McWade, 2016, p. 71), while resilience and recovery are frequently described as "personal" constructs within mental health literature, "certain goals are not permitted. You cannot decide to go to bed or a month". The emphasis on individual efforts and achieving pre-determined therapeutic goals therefore limits the emancipatory potential of resilience discourses for women in mental health settings.

The idea that PTSD only arises in some people following adverse events has also led to a troubling attempt to investigate the traits that allow some people to thrive in the midst of adversity. Such investigations highlight personal deficiency, by arguing that resilience occurs as a result of personal qualities, which are thought to be lacking in people who do not experience post-traumatic growth (Lee, 2017). Their individualistic focus ignores the differing material, social, and symbolic resources that may enable people to be more or less likely to successfully negotiate the effects of significant violence and adversity:

> The fact that some of us seem to survive adverse experience unscathed while others are thrown into confusion or despair may be taken as pointing to "interior", personal qualities: "self-esteem", "willpower", or most recently "resilience". However, it is far easier, and more credible, to point to the embodied advantages someone has acquired over time from the social/material environment than it is to postulate essentially mysterious and unanalysable personal qualities that originate from within.
>
> (The Midlands Psychology Group, 2012, pp. 95–96)

While notions of resilience and growth after violence do provide a welcome reprieve from the problem-saturation of psychiatric constructions of trauma, they are also connected to a broader cultural imperative within neoliberal societies for individuals to manage social forces by being "happy" and "positive" despite adversity (Arts & Van Den Berg, 2018). The happiness imperative has been identified within feminist scholarship as having gendered dimensions, as women are especially reprimanded for expressing fear or anger about their circumstances (Falconer, 2017). Therefore, although the notion of resilience provides some scope for a helpful critique of psychiatric constructions of the symptomatic "traumatised" woman, it offers only a limited refuge from psychiatric oppression, placing responsibilities onto individual women to manage the effects of patriarchal social forces through individual efforts. Consequently, while the potential alignment of notions of resilience to a feminist critique of psychiatric discourses should not be ignored, resilience discourses are also connected to a conservative agenda of expecting mental health service users to manage, accept, and perform optimism in relation to existing norms and power relations.

Concluding reflections

When women speak out about their experiences of gender-based oppression, they have historically run the risk of receiving a barrage of negative responses, ranging from disbelief to victim-blaming and intimidation. Given such hostility, feminist work in mental health on developing a "violence – trauma – symptomatology" narrative is an understandable attempt to create certainty around women's experiences of gendered inequality. However, this chapter has attempted to disrupt the notion that trauma-informed practices offer women an unproblematic pathway towards empowerment and justice. In examining the mainstreaming of the trauma paradigm within mental health services, I have argued that the trauma concept is imbued with a range of meanings, some of which involve a distancing from emancipatory outcomes for women.

The chapter has contended that, in many ways, the trauma concept and related interventions represent a "business-as-usual" approach within psychiatry, whereby women are expected to comply with rigid treatment protocols and accept the advice given by trauma "experts" that they are mentally unstable. In fact, many of the underlying assumptions of trauma theory appear to correspond to the very limitations within conventional psychiatric practices that trauma theory has attempted to critique, for example, pathologising women and femininity, in the absence of a broader social critique of gendered power relations. Therefore, it can be argued that notions of trauma developed by feminist mental health workers and researchers have been appropriated by and subsumed within mainstream mental health discourses in ways that have reduced their transformative possibilities.

However, it would be simplistic and incorrect to claim that the trauma paradigm has completely failed to offer a useful pathway for women to start to reclaim their identities and experiences outside of a biomedical framework. Trauma-informed practices have opened up the possibility for crucial connections to be drawn between women's experiences of distress and violence, alongside other contexts of social inequality. It is necessary, then, to recognise the ways in which the trauma paradigm offers a resource to women who come to the attention of mental health services that is aligned with feminist aims, while also being cautious about its limitations and mixed consequences. A critical analysis of the trauma paradigm continues in Chapter 4, which examines further contestations, including the nexus between trauma and neuroscience discourses and the increasing utilisation of trauma discourses in parenting (mothering) capacity assessments.

References

Ahern, L., & Fisher, D. (2001). Recovery at your own PACE. *Journal of Psychosocial Nursing and Mental Health Services, 39*(4), 22–32.

American Psychiatric Association. (2013). *Diagnostic and statistical manual of mental disorders* (5th ed.). Arlington: American Psychiatric Publishing.

Anonymous. (2018). Will the power threat meaning framework help survivors on welfare? *Asylum: The Magazine for Democratic Psychiatry, 25*, 14.

Arts, J., & Van Den Berg, M. (2018). Pedagogies of optimism: Teaching to 'look forward' in activating welfare programmes in the Netherlands. *Critical Social Policy, online first.* Retrieved from https://doi.org/10.1177/0261018318759923.

Atkinson, J. (2002). *Trauma trails, recreating song lines: The transgenerational effects of trauma in Indigenous Australia.* North Melbourne: Spinifex.

Becker-Blease, K. A. (2017). As the world becomes trauma-informed, work to do. *Journal of Trauma & Dissociation, 18*(2), 131–138.

Behavioral Health Evolution. (2016). *Screening tools help in assessing trauma.* Retrieved from www.bhevolution.org/public/trauma_screening.page.

Bentall, R. P. (2010). *Doctoring the mind: Why psychiatric treatments fail.* London: Penguin Books.

Boler, M. (1997). The risks of empathy: Interrogating multiculturalism's gaze. *Cultural Studies, 11*(2), 253–273.

Bottrell, D. (2009). Understanding 'marginal' perspectives: Towards a social theory of resilience. *Qualitative Social Work, 8*(3), 321–339.

Brandell, J. R. (2004). *Psychodynamic social work.* New York: Columbia University Press.

Briere, J. N. (1992). *Child abuse trauma: Theory and treatment of the lasting effects.* Newbury Park, CA: Sage.

Briere, J., & Jordan, C. E. (2009). Childhood maltreatment, intervening variables, and adult psychological difficulties in women: An overview. *Trauma, Violence and Abuse, 10*(4), 375–388.

Briere, J. N., & Lanktree, C. B. (2012). *Treating complex trauma in adolescents and young adults.* Los Angeles: Sage.

Briere, J. N., & Scott, C. (2015). *Principles of trauma therapy: A guide to symptoms, evaluation, and treatment.* Los Angeles: Sage.

Brock, D. (1991). Talkin' bout a revelation: Feminist popular discourse on sexual abuse. *Canadian Women's Studies, 12*(1), 12–15.

Brown, L. S. (1991). Not outside the range: One feminist perspective on psychic trauma. *American Imago, 48*(1), 119–133.

Brunila, K. (2014). The rise of the survival discourse in an era of therapisation and neoliberalism. *Education Inquiry, 5*(1), 7–23.

Burstow, B. (1992). *Radical feminist therapy: Working in the context of violence.* Newbury Park: Sage.

Burstow, B. (2003). Toward a radical understanding of trauma and trauma work. *Violence Against Women, 9*(11), 1293–1317.

Burstow, B. (2006). Electroshock as a form of violence against women. *Violence Against Women, 12*(4), 372–392.

Caplan, P. (2016). Vets aren't crazy, war is. In W. Hall (Ed.), *Outside mental health: Voices and visions of madness* (pp. 285–286). United States: Madness Radio.

Center for Substance Abuse Treatment. (2014). *Trauma-informed care in behavioral health services. Chapter 4, screening and assessment.* Retrieved from www.ncbi.nlm.nih.gov/books/NBK207188/.

Clarke, K. A., Barnes, M., & Ross, D. (2018). I had no other option: Women, electroconvulsive therapy, and informed consent. *International Journal of Mental Health Nursing, 27*(3), 1077–1085.

Coppock, V., & McGovern, M. (2014). 'Dangerous minds'? Deconstructing counter-terrorism discourse, radicalisation and the 'psychological vulnerability' of muslim children and young people in Britain. *Children & Society, 28*(3), 242–256.

Courtois, C. A. (2004). Complex trauma, complex reactions: Assessment and treatment. *Psychotherapy: Theory, Research, Practice, Training, 41*(4), 412–425.

Cusack, K. J., Frueh, B. C., & Brady, K. T. (2004). Trauma history screening in a community mental health center. *Psychiatric Services, 55*(2), 157–162.

Dillon, J., Johnstone, L., & Longden, E. (2014). Trauma, dissociation, attachment and neuroscience: A new paradigm for understanding severe mental distress. In E. Speed, J. Moncrieff, & M. Rapley (Eds.), *De-medicalizing misery II* (pp. 226–234). London: Palgrave Macmillan.

Elliott, D. E., Bjelajac, P., Fallot, R. D., Markoff, L. S., & Reed, B. G. (2005). Trauma-informed or trauma-denied: Principles and implementation of trauma-informed services for women. *Journal of Community Psychology, 33*(4), 461–477.

Eriksen, K., & Kress, V. E. (2004). *Beyond the DSM story: Ethical quandaries, challenges, and best practices*. Thousand Oaks: Sage.

Esposito, L., & Perez, F. M. (2014). Neoliberalism and the commodification of mental health. *Humanity and Society, 38*(4), 414–442.

Falconer, E. (2017). 'Learning to be Zen': Women travellers and the imperative to happy. *Journal of Gender Studies, 26*(1), 56–65.

Fernandes, S. (2016). *Curated stories: The uses and misuses of storytelling*. New York: Oxford University Press.

Frankel, R. (1998). *The adolescent psyche: Jungian and Winnicottian perspectives*. East Sussex: Routledge.

Friedman, M. J. (2015). *Posttraumatic and acute stress disorders*. Cham: Springer.

Garrett, P. M. (2018). *Welfare words*. London: Sage.

Gavey, N., & Schmidt, J. (2011). "Trauma of rape" discourse: A double-edged template for everyday understandings of the impact of rape? *Violence Against Women, 17*(4), 433–456.

Goodman, R. D. (2013). The transgenerational trauma and resilience genogram. *Counselling Psychology Quarterly, 26*(3–4), 386–405.

Goodman, R. D. (2014). A liberatory approach to trauma counseling: Decolonizing our trauma-informed practices. In R. D. Goodman & P. C. Gorski (Eds.), *Decolonizing 'multicultural' counselling through social justice* (pp. 55–72). New York: Springer.

Haaken, J. (1998). *Pillar of salt: Gender, memory, and the perils of looking back*. New Brunswick: Rutgers University Press.

Hanisch, D., & Moulding, N. (2011). Power, gender and social work responses to child sexual abuse. *Affilia: Journal of Women and Social Work, 26*(3), 278–290.

Harper, D., & Speed, E. (2012). Uncovering recovery: The resistible rise of recovery and resilience. *Studies in Social Justice, 6*(1), 9–25.

Hengehold, L. (2000). Remapping the event: Institutional discourses and the trauma of rape. *Signs: Journal of Women in Culture and society, 26*(1), 189–214.

Herman, J. L. (1992). *Trauma and recovery: The aftermath of violence – From domestic abuse to political terror*. New York: Basic Books.

Hill, M. (1998). Preface. In M. Hill (Ed.), *Feminist therapy as a political act* (pp. xv–xvii). New York: Routledge.

Humphreys, C., & Joseph, S. (2004). Domestic violence and the politics of trauma. *Women's Studies International Quarterly, 27*(5–6), 559–570.

Hunter, N. (2018). *Trauma and madness in mental health services*. New York: Springer.

Johnson, K. (2012). Global mental health, cultural specificity and the risk of neocolonialism: Challenges for critical community psychology. In C. Walker, K. Johnson, & L. Cunningham (Eds.), *Community psychology and the socio-economics of mental distress: International perspectives* (pp. 269–284). Houndmills: Palgrave Macmillan.

Joseph, S., & Linley, P. A. (Eds.). (2008). *Trauma, recovery, and growth: Positive psychological perspectives on posttraumatic stress.* Hoboken, NJ: John Wiley & Sons.

Josewski, V. (2017). A "third space" for doing social justice research. In M. Morrow & L. H. Malcoe (Eds.), *Critical inquiries for social justice in mental health* (pp. 60–86). Toronto: University of Toronto Press.

Kinnucan, M. (2014). *An interview with Yasmin Nair, part two: The ideal neoliberal subject is the subject of trauma.* Retrieved from http://hypocritereader.com/43/yasmin-nair-two.

Kira, I. A., Ashby, J. S., Omidy, A. Z., & Lewandowski, L. (2015). Current, continuous, and cumulative trauma-focused cognitive behavior therapy: A new model for trauma counseling. *Journal of Mental Health Counseling, 37*(4), 323–340.

Knight, C. (2015). Trauma-informed social work practice: Practice considerations and challenges. *Clinical Social Work Journal, 43*(1), 25–37.

Kretschmar, J. M., Butcher, F., Tossone, K., & Beale, B. L. (2016). Examining the concurrent validity of the trauma symptoms checklist for children. *Research on Social Work Practice, 28*(7), 882–890.

Kulkarni, J. (2015). *Borderline personality disorder is a hurtful label for real suffering – Time we changed it.* Retrieved from https://theconversation.com/borderline-personality-disorder-is-a-hurtful-label-for-real-suffering-time-we-changed-it-41760.

Latalova, K., Ociskova, M., Prasko, J., Sedlackova, Z., & Kamaradova, D. (2015). If you label me, go with your therapy somewhere! Borderline personality disorder and stigma. *European Psychiatry, 30*, 1520.

Lee, D. A. (2017). A person-centred political critique of current discourses in post-traumatic stress disorder and post-traumatic growth. *Psychotherapy and Politics International, 15*(2), e1411.

Levenson, J. (2017). Trauma-informed social work practice. *Social Work, 62*(2), 105–113.

Lieb, K., Völlm, B., Rücker, G., Timmer, A., & Stoffers, J. M. (2010). Pharmacotherapy for borderline personality disorder: Cochrane systematic review of randomised trials. *The British Journal of Psychiatry, 196*(1), 4–12.

Linklater, R. (2014). *Decolonizing trauma work.* Halifax: Fernwood Publishing.

Longden, E., Madill, A., & Waterman, M. G. (2012). Dissociation, trauma, and the role of lived experience: Toward a new conceptualization of voice hearing. *Psychological Bulletin, 138*(1), 28–76.

Longden, E., & Read, J. (2016). Social adversity in the etiology of psychosis: A review of the evidence. *American Journal of Psychotherapy, 70*(1), 5–33.

Masson, J. M. (2012). *Against therapy: Emotional tyranny and the myth of psychological healing.* Ebook. Untreed Reads.

Maylea, C. (2016). An end to involuntary treatment in Australian mental health social work. In N. Paul & P. Jones (Eds.), *Social work and health: Inclusive practice research and education* (pp. 94–119). Kerala: Depaul Centre for Research and Development.

McLellan, B. (1995). *Beyond psychoppression.* North Melbourne: Spinifex.

McLeod, J., & Wright, K. (2009). The talking cure in everyday life: Gender, generations and friendship. *Sociology, 43*(1), 122–139.

McWade, B. (2016). Recovery-as-policy as a form of neoliberal state making. *Intersectionalities: A Global Journal of Social Work Analysis, Research, Polity, and Practice, 5*(3), 62–81.

Moloney, P. (2016). Mindfulness: The bottled water of the therapy industry. In R. E. Purser, D. Forbes, & A. Burke (Eds.), *Handbook of mindfulness: Culture, context and social engagement* (pp. 269–292). Cham: Springer.

Moulding, N. (2015). *Gendered violence, abuse and mental health in everyday lives: Beyond trauma*. London: Routledge.

Muskett, C. (2014). Trauma-informed care in inpatient mental health settings: A review of the literature. *International Journal of Mental Health Nursing, 23*(1), 51–59.

Naples, N. A. (2003). Deconstructing and locating survivor discourse: Dynamics of narrative, empowerment, and resistance for survivors of childhood sexual abuse. *Signs: Journal of Women in Culture And Society, 28*(4), 1151–1185.

Nicki, A. (2016). Borderline personality disorder, discrimination, and survivors of chronic childhood trauma. *IJFAB: International Journal of Feminist Approaches to Bioethics, 9*(1), 218–245.

NSW Kids and Families. (2014). *Youth health resource kit: An essential guide for workers*. Sydney: NSW Kids and Families.

O'Brien, W. (2012). The recovery imperative: A critical examination of mid-life women's recovery from depression. *Social Science & Medicine, 75*(3), 573–580.

O'Hagan, M. (2014). *Madness made me*. Wellington: Open Box.

Oudshoorn, J. (2015). *Trauma-informed youth justice: A new framework toward a kinder future*. Toronto: Canadian Scholars' Press.

Pilgrim, D., & McCranie, A. (2013). *Recovery and mental health: A critical sociological account*. Houndmills: Palgrave Macmillan.

Razer, H. (2016). *Writers and artists – Your personal pain is not a blow for justice*. Retrieved from https://dailyreview.com.au/razer-2/43303/.

Recovery in the Bin. (n.d.). *RITB – Key principles*. Retrieved from https://recoveryinthebin.org/ritbkeyprinciples/.

Rees, S., & Fisher, J. (2016). Gender-based violence and women's mental health: How should the GP respond? *Medicine Today, 17*(3), 14–20.

Roberts-Pedersen, E. (2015). *From shell shock to PTSD: Proof of war's traumatic history*. Retrieved from https://theconversation.com/from-shell-shock-to-ptsd-proof-of-wars-traumatic-history-37858.

Rosenthal, M. N., Reinhardt, K. M., & Birrell, P. J. (2016). Guest editorial: Deconstructing disorder: An ordered reaction to a disordered environment. *Journal of Trauma & Dissociation, 17*(2), 131–137.

Ross, D. (2018). A social work perspective on seclusion and restraint in Australia's public mental health system. *Journal of Progressive Human Services, 29*(1), 1–19.

Roy, M., Rivest, M. P., & Moreau, N. (2016). The banality of psychology. *Social Work, 62*(1), 86–88.

Scull, A. (2011). *Madness: A very short introduction*. Oxford: Oxford University Press.

Smail, D. (1996). *How to survive without psychotherapy*. London: Constable.

Smith, M., & Woodiwiss, J. (2016). Sexuality, innocence and agency in narratives of childhood sexual abuse: Implications for social work. *The British Journal of Social Work, 46*(8), 2173–2189.

Swan, E. (2008). 'You make me feel like a woman': Therapeutic cultures and the contagion of femininity. *Gender, Work & Organization, 15*(1), 88–107.

Sweeney, A., Clement, S., Filson, B., & Kennedy, A. (2016). Trauma-informed mental healthcare in the UK: What is it and how can we further its development? *Mental Health Review Journal, 21*(3), 174–192.

Taft, A. (2003). *Promoting women's mental health: The challenges of intimate partner/domestic violence* (Issues Paper 8). Australian Domestic and Family Violence Clearinghouse. Retrieved from www.austdvclearinghouse.unsw.edu.au/PDF%20files/Issues_Paper_8.pdf.

The Midlands Psychology Group. (2012). Draft manifesto for a social materialist psychology of distress. *Journal of Critical Psychology, Counselling and Psychotherapy, 12*(2), 93–107.

The National Child Traumatic Stress Network. (n.d.). *Screening and assessment.* Retrieved from www.nctsn.org/what-is-child-trauma/trauma-types/complex-trauma/screening-and-assessment.

Todd, N., Wade, A., & Renoux, M. (2004). Coming to terms with violence and resistance. In *Furthering talk* (pp. 145–161). Boston: Springer.

Trevillion, K., Corker, E., Capron, L. E., & Oram, S. (2016). Improving mental health service responses to domestic violence and abuse. *International Review of Psychiatry, 28*(5), 423–432.

Ungar, M. (2011). The social ecology of resilience: Addressing contextual and cultural ambiguity of a nascent construct. *American Journal of Orthopsychiatry, 81*(1), 1–17.

Ussher, J. M. (2013). Diagnosing difficult women and pathologising femininity: Gender bias in psychiatric nosology. *Feminism & Psychology, 23*(1), 63–69.

van Daalen-Smith, C., Adam, S., Breggin, P., & LeFrançois, B. A. (2014). The utmost discretion: How presumed prudence leaves children susceptible to electroshock. *Children & Society, 28*(3), 205–217.

Van der Kolk, B. A. (2017). Developmental trauma disorder: Toward a rational diagnosis for children with complex trauma histories. *Psychiatric Annals, 35*(5), 401–408.

Wade, A. (1997). Small acts of living: Everyday resistance to violence and other forms of oppression. *Contemporary Family Therapy, 19*(1), 23–39.

Wade, A. (2014). *Response-based practice with victims of violence.* Retrieved from www.womenscouncil.com.au/uploads/6/1/1/9/6119703/rbp_101.pdf.

Wagner, A. W., & Linehan, M. M. (1994). Relationship between childhood sexual abuse and topography of parasuicide among women with borderline personality disorder. *Journal of Personality Disorders, 8*(1), 1–9.

Wallcraft, J., & Hopper, K. (2015). The capabilities approach and the social model of mental health. In H. Spandler, J. Anderson, & B. Sapey (Eds.), *Madness, distress and the politics of disablement* (pp. 83–98). Bristol: The Policy Press.

White, M. (1995). *Re-authoring lives: Interviews and essays.* Adelaide: Dulwich Centre Publications.

Wright, K. (2008). Theorizing therapeutic culture: Past influences, future directions. *Journal of Sociology, 44*(4), 321–336.

Zhang, H. (2017). How 'anti-ing' becomes mastery: Moral subjectivities shaped through anti-oppressive practice. *British Journal of Social Work, 48*(1), 124–140.

4 Symptoms or social justice? Contested understandings of trauma

The previous chapter provided a critical analysis of the trauma paradigm's influence in contemporary mental health services, commencing with a discussion of the potential alignment of trauma-informed practices with feminist critiques of biomedical psychiatry. It discussed arguments made by proponents of the trauma paradigm that the trauma concept opens up a radically different framework for mental health service provision, which is empowering, woman-centred, and interested in the links between mental health presentations and systemic issues of gender inequality and violence. On the other hand, a more critical approach to trauma has demonstrated the many ways in which the trauma concept mirrors a conventional psychiatric intervention, by retaining a deficit-lens, inviting a standardised therapeutic response, and minimising power relations present both within gender-based violence and mental health interventions. This chapter continues a critical analysis of trauma-informed ideas and their implications for women, through an examination of two growing areas of interest relating to the trauma paradigm: the study of the brain-based effects of violence, where neuroscience data is used to support claims about trauma; and an exploration of nexus between trauma symptomatology and diminished "mothering capacity". The emphasis placed within these research agendas on women's symptomatology after violence suggest an increasingly narrow scope for feminist activism within trauma discourses. The chapter concludes with a discussion about the increasingly broad use of the trauma concept, whereby the diverse iterations of the trauma paradigm mean that it is no longer possible to refer to trauma as a single concept. As a result, it is necessary to critically analyse claims relating to trauma and trauma-informed practices, interrogating their varying socio-political underpinnings and implications.

Neuroscience and trauma

In Chapter 2, I outlined concerns raised by critical mental health scholars about the biological determinism involved in mainstream psychiatric discourses, especially the notion that mental distress occurs as a result of brain dysfunctions or neurochemical imbalances – an idea that continues to enjoy widespread influence, despite increasing concerns about its tenuous evidence base. Despite the trauma paradigm's focus on the interpersonal and social causes of distress, trauma research has nonetheless shown a strong willingness to engage with neurobiological discourses in developing knowledge about the effects of violence and abuse. Advocates of trauma-informed mental health practices have attempted to use neurobiology to demonstrate the brain impairments that can be seen in women and children in the aftermath of violence, and trauma research is often heavily imbued with neurobiological ideas:

> We have used PET to study neural circuits of trauma-related disorders in women with early abuse and a variety of trauma spectrum mental disorders. . . . Women with abuse and PTSD showed a failure of hippocampal activation during the memory task relative to controls. Women with abuse and PTSD in this study also had smaller hippocampal volume measured with MRI relative to both women with abuse without PTSD and non-abused non-PTSD women.
>
> (Bremner, 2006, p. 451)

As well as in academic journals, research into the brain-based effects of trauma have been widely reported within popular media contexts:

> Several in-depth studies, using neuroimaging technology to map the brains of PTSD sufferers, have been conducted. These have outlined dramatic changes in brain structures and functions. The three most impacted places are the amygdala, the hippocampus, and the ventromedial prefrontal cortex (vmPFC). These complete the stress circuit inside the brain, and are responsible for the symptoms a sufferer continues to experience.
>
> (Big Think, 2018, n.p.)

Feminists have largely embraced the role of neuroscience within trauma research, and for understandable reasons: neuroscientific discourses have reached a position of immense esteem and prominence within the global north, with the result being an era of "neuroenchantment" (Ali, Lifshitz, & Raz, 2014). The allure of neuroscience reflects an increasing preoccupation within highly medicalised societies with brain processes, based on the notion that the brain is the location of the "modern self" (Vidal, 2009). Consequently, "brain claims" are often met with excitement and at times an undue lack of caution regarding their relevance to an ever-increasing range of social policy areas (Macvarish, Lee, & Lowe, 2014). Neuro-discourses are drawn upon in the context of trauma-informed practice to add weight to the claim that gender-based violence is a serious issue, with immense consequences for women and children that cannot be trivialised:

> the present study provides evidence for the neuroanatomical injury associated with self-blame attributions, and emphasizes the need for a change in current social stand [sic] toward sexually assaulted individuals.
>
> (Berman, Assaf, Tarrasch, & Joel, 2018, p. 8)

Neuroscience discourses are therefore useful in opening up avenues for examining the effects of trauma on women's lives that offer a sharp counterpoint to patriarchal discourses of victim-blaming, denial, or minimisation that continue to shape the responses that women receive when disclosing experiences of gender-based violence. Although the scientific evidence for the impact of violence on brains is in its very early stages, neuro-knowledges have garnered significant influence within both the public imagination and professional contexts in shaping how the effects of violence (among other major stressors and oppressions) are understood. Despite the influence and wide acceptance of Herman's (1992) conceptualisation of trauma, her analysis has been linked to neurobiological evidence as a strategy to strengthen the perceived veracity of her claims:

> Herman's concept of "terror" can now be described as the nervous system's reaction to trauma . . . the student of neurobiology can observe how Herman's work laid the groundwork that described how PTSD activates the hypothalamic-pituitary-adrenocortical (HPA)-axis's response to trauma. The HPA-axis is responsible for the "physiological homeostasis". . . . A severely traumatized client has become calibrated to sustain high levels of HPA-axis activation and sympathetic nervous system arousal.
>
> (Zaleski, Johnson, & Klein, 2016, p. 381)

In this way, neuroscience discourses have been drawn upon by some feminist and critical mental health workers as a form of advocacy in highlighting the significance of gender-based oppressions in shaping women's experiences of distress. Neuroscience discourses add scientific authority to claims made about women's distress following violence, seemingly ending decades of societal disregard for feminist concerns about the pervasive problem of gender-based violence and a vastly under-funded feminist agenda aimed at addressing violence against women. There are, however, a number of troubling implications involved in the enactment of neuro-knowledges as a strategy of feminist activism, as neuroscience evidence is used for other more conservative or individualising aims. For example, neuro-imaging techniques are drawn upon to measure the effectiveness of trauma-based mental health interventions following gender-based violence and other adverse events, providing them with a stamp of scientific certainty (for example, Boyd, Lanius, & McKinnon, 2018). Also troubling is the use of neuro-imaging techniques to make claims about pre-existing vulnerabilities within the brains of women who have been diagnosed with PTSD in response to adverse events:

> [E]merging evidence suggests that the final PTSD pathology results from both predisposed and acquired neural abnormalities. In particular, when analysing between-group differences in neural activity for PTSD compared to healthy controls, it is often unclear whether such functional differences correspond to pre-existing vulnerabilities.
>
> (Stark et al., 2015)

Such claims shift the focus away from the effects of the adverse experiences, towards an exploration of the biological factors that have caused a susceptibility to trauma symptoms. The investigation into the brain-based causes of women's distress following adverse events seems perilously close to a mainstream bio-medical preoccupation with women's internal dysfunctions as a cause of mental illness (Lee, 2017). Thus, while trauma discourses promise to circumvent biological determinism, the increasing reliance on neuroscience data means that they are at times involved in narrow analyses of women's symptoms and brains, leaving little space for a social analysis.

Although the harm resulting from violence can be measured in a variety of ways, including listening to women's accounts of their own experiences, and observing or getting to know a person, the "seductive allure" of neuroscience within contemporary societies means that neuroimaging is positioned as producing more reliable or weighty evidence than narrative or behavioural explorations (Fine, 2010, p. 169). This elevation of neuro-knowledges above other forms of research has been in part a pragmatic strategy by feminist mental health workers and researchers that has attempted to locate violence against women as a serious issue that poses significant harm to women and children's lives. However, such engagements come at the substantial cost of de-centring women's voices, invisibilising a diversity of experiences among women, with the result being a conferral of expertise – once again – to medical professionals. In emphasising biological processes, neuro-knowledges engage in the very reductionism that the trauma paradigm claims to reject: trauma is constructed as a biological deviation, for medical professionals to treat, whereby the socio-political contexts that have given rise to women's experiences of violence are set aside in favour of a treatment response based upon "fixing" women.

Other neuroscientific discourses on trauma appear to offer far more optimistic accounts. For example, some researchers have emphasised that while brain impairments may arise through exposure to abuse and violence, these detrimental changes can be reversed and repaired. Referred to as neuroplasticity, processes of brain repair following adverse events are believed to include the development of new brain cells and new synaptic connections, and the weakening of other synaptic connections (Pitts-Taylor, 2010). Upon first glance, the notion of neuroplasticity seems to provide a reprieve from the deficit-orientation and determinism that are present within both conventional mental health discourses and trauma discourses. Notions of neuroplasticity have given rise to a hope-filled research agenda exploring the social and environmental factors that are important in supporting this repair work (Combs-Orme, 2017). Nevertheless, more critical analyses of neuroplasticity have argued that their seemingly more optimistic stance is not necessarily any more capable of leading to women's empowerment than is the traditional narrative of brain dysfunction. Rather, neuroplasticity plays neatly into a self-management discourse whereby women are positioned as responsible for achieving good outcomes and recovery after trauma, even in the absence of any resources to do so (Pitts-Taylor, 2010). Narratives of dysfunction and narratives of neuroplasticity following violence provide contradictory messages about the effects of trauma: at the same time that women are advised that they will experience long-term psychological deficiencies due to the effects of trauma on brains, they are advised of the brain's astonishing capacity to recover. While some writers contend that deterministic neuro-discourses are replacing psychological self-management discourses as a dominant framework for understanding human experience, Rose and Abi-Rached (2013) conversely argue that the contradictions between neurobiological understandings and psychological discourses result in a multiple repertoire of the self, whereby neurobiological processes are privileged and yet seen as adaptable through individual efforts. The following excerpt demonstrates this convergence of neurobiological determinism and self-management ideas:

> Biofeedback is a range of techniques to gain voluntary control of physiological functions, which are normally regulated without conscious awareness. By tapping into these physiological functions you can take control of your body rather than being controlled by it.
>
> (Neuro Resilience, n.d.)

The disconnect between notions of dysfunction and neuroplasticity mirror the inconsistencies or "mixed messages" within contemporary constructions of femininity, for example, pressures on women to fulfil traditional feminine roles, while also exercising autonomy (for example, through building a career) – with a "no win" or "damned if you do, damned if you don't" outcome for women (Moulding, 2017). The interview data presented in Chapter 5 further exemplify the contradictory expectations placed upon women after violence, wherein women discussed how they were placed under pressure to accept the construction of a "damaged" self in the aftermath of violence, but also to actively engage in strategies to moderate the effects of abuse through taxing therapy and self-management strategies.

In concluding this discussion on neuroscience, it would be remiss not to mention that the exaggerated and premature claims of neuroscience have been documented by both sociologists and neuroscientists themselves (Fine, 2010; Rose & Abi-Rached, 2013). A pertinent example is the now almost ubiquitous notion that infant brains can be distinguished from adult brains by rapid growth and developmental processes that occur in very young children. This notion has led to the idea that there is an extremely narrow window of opportunity to provide children with the learning and relational opportunities that are necessary for successful adulthood, meaning that experiences of early abuse are viewed as causing irreparable and pervasive damage – a discourse that has been named the "first three years movement", which has enjoyed pervasive influence on social policy, human service practice, and academic research agenda (Garrett, 2017). The infant determinism that is embedded in this claim has been challenged on a number of grounds, including its heavy reliance on data from animal studies; the use of data gathered from extreme cases of abuse, which are presumed to be relevant to situations of lesser abuse; and a lack of acknowledgement of evidence suggesting the large capacity of adults for learning (Bruer, 2002; Derbyshire, 2011).

As neuro-knowledges are being afforded an ever-increasing status and growing influence within human service contexts, a critical analysis of their use in the area of trauma-informed mental health practices is now urgently required. While it is important to avoid a stance that stubbornly rejects all neuroscientific knowledge within an interdisciplinary approach to feminism and the study of trauma, its contribution must be appropriately weighted and read carefully. For example, simple yet remarkably common errors such as believing that colourful neuroscience images are "pictures" of the brain and brain activity, instead of representations of statistical data, demonstrate an overzealous and clumsy use of neuroscience data (Fine, 2010). Such practices invite the unwarranted scrutiny of individual women following experiences of violence, with socio-political analyses neglected in favour of a treatment response.

A "traumatised mothering" discourse

In the past two decades, an extensive body of psychological research has emerged regarding the nexus between maternal experiences of abuse, trauma symptomatology, and mothering "capacity". In view of the overwhelmingly problem-saturated literature on motherhood in the context of mental illness, the utilisation of the trauma concept within parenting assessments is a particularly pertinent area for feminist investigation. Within human service contexts and beyond, mothers with mental illness diagnoses have historically been constructed as dangerous and ineffective parents, with a range of problematic behaviours including being self-preoccupied, emotionally withdrawn, and unpredictable, to name but a few examples, and such constructions continue into a contemporary context (Halsa, 2018). It is worthwhile to explore, then, the effect that trauma discourses have had on the construction of mothers and mothering within mental health settings. Given that trauma-informed practices claim to offer empowering, holistic, and contextualised understandings of women's lives in comparison to psychiatric discourses, does the deployment of the trauma paradigm lead to more empowering, holistic, and contextualised understandings of women and mothering?

Unfortunately, research in the area of trauma and parenting capacity appears to be largely concerned with the continuation of a dominant narrative about mental distress leading to harmful mothering practices. The literature documents wide-ranging concerns about the effects of maternal violence-related PTSD stemming from mothers' exposure to gender-based violence both in childhood and adulthood, for example:

- The harmful effects of maternal abuse history and PTSD on "negative attributions" towards their children:

  [W]ithin a non-referred community paediatrics clinic sample, the severity of mothers' trauma-related psychopathology, in particular, their interpersonal violence-related (IPV) post-traumatic stress, dissociative, and depressive symptoms predicted the degree of negativity of mothers' attributions towards their preschool age children, themselves, and their own primary attachment figure (Schechter et al., 2015, p. 10).

- The harmful effects of maternal abuse history and PTSD on parent-child attachment difficulties:

  [D]uring a 6-month postpartum home visit, mothers and infants participated in a dyadic play interaction subsequently coded for positive parenting behaviours by blinded coders . . . women with postpartum psychopathology (depression and post-traumatic stress disorder [PTSD]) showed consistently greater bonding impairment scores at all timepoints. . . . These results highlight the adverse effects of maternal postpartum depression and PTSD on mother-infant bonding in early postpartum in women with child abuse and neglect histories (Muzik et al., 2013, p. 29).

- The harmful effects of maternal experiences of early-life maltreatment on their "sensitivity" during their interactions with their children (a connection that is further solidified through the use of neurobiological data):

  Mothers with early-life maltreatment were less sensitive in real-life mother – child interactions, but while imagining conflictual interactions with their child, they showed increased activation in regions of the salience and emotion-processing network, such as the amygdala, insula and hippocampus. This activation pattern was in contrast to that of mothers without early-life maltreatment (Neukel et al., 2018, p. 272).

The overwhelmingly negative and pathologising tone of the literature on mothering in the aftermath of violence is striking and yet unsurprising. Its deficit-ridden view reflects a widespread cultural trope of mothering, wherein mothers are considered to be a central source of difficulties for their children whenever problems emerge (Jackson & Mannix, 2004). Psychological theories have a long history of constructing mothers as "the disorderly matter that must be sorted out, assembled and disassembled, bonded and broken down" (Adams, 1995, p. 427). The surveillance of mothering in the studies cited above demonstrates a willingness to participate in these long-standing practices of mother-blaming. Notions of children's rapidly developing brains and "critical" periods of infant brain development add layers of perceived objectivity and urgency to this research agenda (Wastell & White, 2012). Demonstrating a collusion with patriarchal conceptualisations of mothering that place a far greater responsibility for parenting and child welfare on women in comparison to men, the studies place unwarranted emphasis on the mother-child dyad, concealing a myriad of other factors that shape children's lives.

Indeed, the literature on trauma and parenting capacity is decidedly gendered in its approach, centring on an assessment of women's behaviours, by often choosing only to examine maternal life histories, maternal psychological functioning, mothering capacity, and child outcomes, and the correlations that can be found between these, with often no acknowledgement of the social, political, and cultural contexts in which parenting occurs. The absence of these broader factors from the analyses results in a disproportionate scrutiny of women's moods, interactions, and behaviours, at the expense of an analysis of the gender and power relations that underpin women's experiences as mothers, alongside other intersections of power, including class and "race". Of course, it also neatly sidesteps the role played by men in child wellbeing and family life, which may be characterised by chronic neglect, or violence and abuse (Heward-Belle, 2016). This is a particularly pertinent issue if women are assessed to have been traumatised through a context of domestic violence. A remarkable erasure in much of this literature is the common tactic utilised by perpetrators of domestic violence to undermine the relationships between mothers and their children (Humphreys, 2011). Furthermore, women living with domestic violence may protect their children in ways that are not recognised by mainstream attachment theory (Buchanan, 2018). Clearly, this dynamic provides much-needed contextual information to sit alongside a simplistic discussion about women, trauma, and mother-child interactions. Therefore, the utilisation of the trauma concept within parenting capacity research provides yet another means of perpetuating already well-established practices of mother-blaming and the disproportionate surveillance of motherhood within the human service sector.

The flourishing area of trauma and attachment theory is particularly striking, given that feminism has been one of attachment theory's strongest critics. Feminist analyses have demonstrated the ways in which attachment theory has been used to oppress women through inviting surveillance of mothering practices as "one of the most enduring discourses aimed at explaining and defining normal (and hence normative) maternal and child roles in the last century" (Thornton in Garrett, 2017, p. 670). By claiming universal relevance, attachment theory perpetuates patriarchal, classist, and Eurocentric values that ignore an array of cross-cultural variations in caregiving practices, including the historical and cultural specificity of so-called "secure" attachment (Gaskins, 2013). The measurement of attachment through observation of mother-child interactions has also been critiqued for positioning women as fundamentally responsible for children's wellbeing, while other caregivers (including fathers) are invisibilised, and social factors and resources are rendered irrelevant (Birns, 1999).

Importantly, it is not the aim of this discussion to dismiss the challenges involved in a consideration of women's capacities to parent after experiencing violence or abuse, nor to deny that such experiences have the capacity to impact negatively on mothering. However, it has attempted to highlight the frequently overlooked need to attend to the impact of gendered power relations on women's lives when considering questions relating to mothering. To do this, it is necessary to critique de-contextualised notions of parenting capacities that pay no attention to the social contexts and resources that are fundamental to understanding children's wellbeing. Furthermore, some of the constructs that women are being assessed against within the "traumatised mothering" research agenda – for example, attachment – have been criticised by feminists as inherently problematic concepts, due to their classed, Eurocentric, and patriarchal assumptions. There is, moreover, a need for an interrogation within the research of the conflation of "parenting" with "mothering"; the lack of consideration of fathers and fathering, and the lack of attention given to children's broader social worlds beyond the mother-child dyad. Engaging with these questions does not mean that women should not be held at all responsible for the welfare of their children. However, it does involve a recognition that mothering occurs within a context of gendered power relations, which may place limitations on the range of possible courses of action that are available to women, as a result of the behaviours of men (Wendt, 2015). It also involves an acknowledgement of the ways in which parenting capacity assessments are not based upon objective and incontestable measurements, but are themselves imbued with a range of biases and assumptions.

The research studies cited above demonstrate how the trauma concept can be utilised in such a way as to be disadvantageous to women's empowerment, leading to deficit-laden, individualising, and de-politicised accounts of women's lives following violence. In stark contrast to feminist theory and values, constructions of "traumatised mothers" risk re-inscribing psychiatric notions of women's dysfunction, while placing the responsibility on women to manage the effects of gender-based violence. The notion of "traumatised mothering" encourages the use of a deterministic narrative for understanding women's experiences after violence, leaving women who disclose a history of abuse within a human service context vulnerable to pre-emptive assumptions being made about their parenting capacities. Far from empowering, such responses may lead to interventions that are inadequately attuned to women's current circumstances and that too readily dismiss the socio-political contexts in which mothering is constructed, performed, and assessed.

Genericising trauma

As trauma-informed practices have moved from the peripheries of mental health care to take an increasingly central position, there have been concerns raised about the risk of trauma becoming a nebulous idea:

> While such efforts to create more effective service systems are laudable, TIC [trauma-informed care] is an amorphous concept. . . . *Trauma informed* has become a standard term in our nomenclature and yet there does not appear to be a clear consensus on what TIC actually means nor delineation of the specific components needed to achieve it.
>
> (Hanson & Lang, 2016, p. 96, italics in original)

Despite efforts to differentiate between single episode events and complex trauma arising from chronic and interpersonal acts of violence, the trauma concept is now regularly invoked to describe the effects of such wide-ranging events as motor vehicle accidents, natural disasters, bullying, poverty, chronic illness, divorce, among other adverse experiences. At the same time, trauma has become a culturally salient concept within the global north, wherein trauma is thought to speak to an essential and timeless "truth" about the universal human condition (Bracken, 2002). Ideas about the supposed universality of trauma are evident within contemporary re-readings of texts claiming, for example, that the works of Homer, Shakespeare and Dickens portray characters who are affected by trauma, despite little or no mention of it (Friedman, 2015). Given the salience of the trauma concept and its capacity to add legitimacy to narratives of distress, an inclusive and expansive approach to trauma is an understandable attempt to avoid the creation of a hierarchy of despair, wherein only certain distressing experiences are understood to be traumatic. Nevertheless, the professional interests that are served by increasing the perceived relevance and scope for therapeutic trauma interventions should also be recognised (Naples, 2003). A result of the generic use of the trauma concept is a grouping together of experiences with very little in common, leaving limited opportunity for their varying socio-political contexts to be differentiated, and with a very strong focus instead being placed on trauma symptoms and treatment-focused concerns. Kirmayer, Gone, and Moses (2014, p. 313) note the political dangerousness of conflating disparate forms of violence under notions of trauma, as "specific historical wrongs require their own modes of understanding and have their own moral imperatives". Given that a major aim of trauma-informed practices relating to gender-based violence was the elevation of women's voices and a critique of the psychiatric colonising of women's experiences, the ever-increasing scope of the term "trauma" is concerning. In an attempt to expand the perceived relevance of trauma-informed perspectives, trauma has been described as a universal human experience to which the majority of the population is exposed at some point during their lives (Black Dog Institute, 2017). Such all-encompassing claims about trauma risk diluting the capacity of the trauma paradigm to respond to the specificity of women's concerns about gender-based violence and muting robust feminist perspectives relating to patriarchal experience.

The relevance of trauma-informed principles are now seemingly ubiquitous, arising in an increasingly vast range of settings beyond mental health, for example, in dentistry, where professionals are advised to take more care in consent processes before embarking on treatment (Raja, Hoersch, Rajagopalan, & Chang, 2014). The generic nature of trauma-informed practices means that they are thought to be beneficial for people with or without experiences that could be classed as traumatic (Elliott, Bjelajac, Fallot, Markoff, & Reed, 2005). Muskett's (2014, p. 58) review of literature on trauma-informed approaches in mental health settings concluded that trauma-informed care broadly refers to "the use of strategies that most would consider basic ingredients of contemporary, effective mental health care", with some versions of trauma-informed practice involving strategies that are as simple as the adoption of a respectful manner. It is noteworthy that most of the guidelines of trauma-informed services – the importance of trustworthiness, choice, collaboration and empowerment – are not novel principles, but in fact underpin a broad range of therapeutic approaches that were in existence prior to the proliferation of the trauma concept. Trauma-informed practices are not always grounded in a political commitment to analysing issues of power, gender inequality, and other forms of oppression. When the link between feminist activism and trauma is lost, the question of whether there is any meaningful difference between a trauma-informed perspective and a conventional approach to mental health service provision is open to question. Moreover, some of the examples described in this chapter show the trauma concept being used in ways that invite oppressive and patriarchal understandings of women's experiences.

Elsewhere, I have reported on empirical research into professional constructions of abuse and trauma within the context of child and adolescent mental health services (Tseris, 2018). Within this research, the trauma concept did not provide a unifying framework to assist social workers in understanding young women's mental health presentations, but rather, notions of trauma were used for a variety of purposes: to diagnose women with mental health issues; to predict lifelong psychological and interpersonal problems; to implement rigid therapeutic strategies; or to speak with young women about gender inequality and its effects on their lives. Consequently, I argued that the trauma paradigm is best understood as an "umbrella concept" with a number of divergent iterations, meaning that:

> it is possible to use the trauma concept in a variety of ways, and that not all trauma work with female survivors of violence incorporates an analysis of gendered power relations, the privileging of social contexts, or the de-centering of therapeutic expertise.
>
> (Tseris, 2018, p. 16)

An approach to trauma work that focuses on the problematic characteristics of women after abuse is likely to be connected to the expansion of mainstream mental health service provision as a dominant response to violence, leading to increases in diagnosis, medication prescription, and one-on-one work therapeutic work with service users, at the expense of other more systemic responses (Rimke & Brock, 2012). An approach of this kind was evident among participants who described the complex symptomotology of service users after violence and who positioned themselves as playing an expert role in attempting to diminish their distress. This can be contrasted with a more politicised analysis of distress, which could incorporate the need for alternatives to clinical and one-on-one support for women in the aftermath of abuse, adopting a wider lens that examines material needs, deconstructs dominant medical discourses of mental health, and considers the benefits of community work, education, and grassroots activism (Karban, 2017). However, there was an absence of responses other than therapy within the majority of interviews and most participants' agency contexts offered very limited support for activist work or community engagement.

The diverse utilisation of trauma-informed practices by social workers reflects social work's complex relationship to psychiatric and therapeutic discourses, as an explicitly critical profession with specific training in sociology. Social work is therefore able to articulate the limited capacity of psychiatric knowledge in explaining the social context, consequences, and causes of mental illness (Fawcett, 2012). Additionally, social work practice is characterised by an espoused acceptance of uncertainty, ambiguity, and tensions, with Fook (2013, p. 29) going so far as to suggest that uncertainty is perhaps the "defining characteristic" of social work. This stance contrasts with the often inflexible diagnostic approach of psychiatry and its reliance on certain types of evidence that increase levels of perceived certainty when working with service users. Nevertheless, the extent to which social work genuinely engages with uncertainty is contestable, and perhaps excessively emphasised (White, 2009), and many social workers routinely draw upon the DSM to inform their work, despite its assumptions about internal pathologies conflicting with social work values and principles including collaboration with service users and naming social inequalities (Frances & Jones, 2014; Kirk & Kutchins, 1992). Social workers are also confronted with risk discourses in their everyday work in mental health services, which in many ways run counter to social work's acknowledgement of power relations and social inequalities. Discourses of risk contain highly pathologising understandings of service users as dangerous individuals, leading to defensive practices aimed at controlling service users' behaviours while ignoring structural disadvantage (Stanford, 2010). Contemporary domains of social work practice include cognitive behavioural therapy (Neal, Jackson, & McDermott, 2014) and private practice (Ftanoua et al., 2014), demonstrating that social work is at times left struggling to articulate a sociological perspective on mental health, instead reproducing psychiatric and individualistic discourses. Social work has been accused of forming an allegiance with psychiatric practices as a way of increasing the power and status of the profession (Gomery, Wong, Cohen, & Lacasse, 2011). Although such clashing agendas are acute within social work contexts, other non-psychiatric mental health disciplines face similar challenges as they attempt to hold the sometimes contradictory contributions of sociological and clinical knowledges in tension. As noted by Godard and Josewski (2017, pp. 434–435), the trauma concept has multiple meanings and implications: "a narrow focus on trauma omits women's experiences of systemic oppression and structural violence", however when an emphasis is placed on structural rather than private explanations, trauma-informed practice "situates women's experiences of violence within multiple oppressions and highlights perpetrator and systemic social accountability". The breadth of the trauma concept means that it is open to an increasingly vast range of interpretations, and feminist scholars and human service workers alike must be vigilant about its multiple iterations.

Concluding reflections

Alongside Chapter 3, this chapter has offered a critical analysis of the multiple iterations of the trauma paradigm – both its potential to support emancipatory work with women, as well as the more troubling finding that trauma work can be taken up in ways that are misaligned with the social justice principles that the trauma paradigm purports to promote. The breadth and slipperiness of the trauma concept allow for multiple interpretations and, consequently, trauma is an increasingly nebulous concept. Troublingly, this chapter has provided a number of poignant examples of the trauma concept being utilised in ways that support deficit-laden and de-politicised views of women's lives following violence, and invite new forms of surveillance and assessment. The increasing focus on pre-disposing factors for PTSD within individual women alongside an emphasis on neurobiological processes demonstrates the potential for the trauma paradigm to become no more than "a rhetorical device for retaining the primacy of biological factors . . . reducing life events to the status of 'trigger' for an underlying disease process" (Dillon, Johnstone, & Longden, 2014, p. 232). Having outlined a num-ber of concerns relating to the contemporary uptake of trauma in mental health settings, Chapter 5 turns to empirical work involving the perspectives of women with experiences of gender-based violence during their adolescence. Their per-spectives on medicalised and therapeutic practices demonstrate further both the possibilities and hazards of the trauma paradigm as a way of understanding the problem of violence against women.

References

Adams, A. (1995). Maternal bonds: Recent literature on mothering. *Signs: Journal of Women in Culture and Society, 20*(2), 414–427.

Ali, S. S., Lifshitz, M., & Raz, A. (2014). Empirical neuroenchantment: From reading minds to thinking critically. *Frontiers in Human Neuroscience, 8,* 357.

Berman, Z., Assaf, Y., Tarrasch, R., & Joel, D. (2018). Assault-related self-blame and its association with PTSD in sexually assaulted women: An MRI inquiry. *Social Cognitive and Affective Neuroscience, online first.* doi: 10.1093/scan/nsy044.

Big Think. (2018). *Been traumatized? Here's how PTSD rewires the brain.* Retrieved from https://bigthink.com/philip-perry/been-traumatized-here-is-how-ptsd-rewires-the-brain.

Birns, B. (1999). Attachment theory revisited: Challenging conceptual and methodological sacred cows. *Feminism & Psychology, 9*(1), 10–21.

Black Dog Institute. (2017). *Trauma and mental health.* Retrieved from www.blackdog institute.org.au/research/key-research-areas/trauma-and-mental-health.

Boyd, J. E., Lanius, R. A., & McKinnon, M. C. (2018). Mindfulness-based treatments for posttraumatic stress disorder: A review of the treatment literature and neurobiological evidence. *Journal of Psychiatry & Neuroscience: JPN, 43*(1), 7.

Bracken, P. (2002). *Trauma: Culture, meaning and philosophy.* Philadelphia: Whurr Publishers.

Bremner, J. D. (2006). Traumatic stress: Effects on the brain. *Dialogues in Clinical Neu-roscience, 8*(4), 445–461.

Bruer, J. (2002). *The myth of the first three years.* New York: The Free Press.

Buchanan, F. (2018). *Mothering babies in domestic violence: Beyond attachment theory.* Abingdon: Routledge.

Combs-Orme, T. (2017). Epigenetics revisioned: Reply to white and wastell. *British Jour-nal of Social Work, 48*(2), 531–535.

Derbyshire, S. W. G. (2011). *The problem of infant neurodeterminism.* Paper presented at the Monitoring Parents: Science, Evidence, Experts and the New Parenting Culture. Retrieved from http://blogs.kent.ac.uk/parentingculturestudies/fles/2011/09/Stuart-Derbyshire_2011.pdf.

Dillon, J., Johnstone, L., & Longden, E. (2014). Trauma, dissociation, attachment and neuroscience: A new paradigm for understanding severe mental distress. In E. Speed,

J. Moncrieff, & M. Rapley (Eds.), *De-medicalizing misery II* (pp. 226–234). London: Palgrave Macmillan.

Elliott, D. E., Bjelajac, P., Fallot, R. D., Markoff, L. S., & Reed, B. G. (2005). Trauma-informed or trauma-denied: Principles and implementation of trauma-informed services for women. *Journal of Community Psychology, 33*(4), 461–477.

Fawcett, B. (2012). Mental health. In M. Gray, J. Midgley, & S. A. Webb (Eds.), *Sage handbook of social work*. London: Sage.

Fine, C. (2010). *Delusions of gender*. Duxford: Icon Books.

Fook, J. (2013). Uncertainty: The defining characteristic of social work? In V. E. Cree (Ed.), *Social work: A reader* (pp. 29–34). Oxon: Routledge.

Frances, A., & Jones, K. D. (2014). Should social workers use *diagnostic and statistical manual of mental disoders-5? Research on Social Work Practice, 24*(1), 11–12.

Friedman, M. J. (2015). *Posttraumatic and acute stress disorders*. Cham: Springer.

Ftanoua, M., Williamsona, M., Machlina, A., Warra, D., Christoa, J., Castana, L., Harris, M., Bassilios, B. & Pirkisa, J. (2014). Evaluating the better access initiative: What do consumers have to say? *Australian Social Work, 67*(2), 162–168.

Garrett, P. M. (2017). Wired: Early intervention and the 'neuromolecular gaze'. *British Journal of Social Work, 48*(3), 656–674.

Gaskins, S. (2013). The puzzle of attachment: Unscrambling maturational and cultural contributions to the development of early emotional bonds. In N. Quinn & J. Mageo (Eds.), *Attachment reconsidered* (pp. 33–64). New York: Palgrave Macmillan.

Godard, L., & Josewski, V. (2017). Disrupting dominant discourses: Rethinking services and systems for women with experiences of abuse. In M. Morrow & L. H. Malcoe (Eds.), *Critical inquiries for social justice in mental health*. Toronto: University of Toronto Press.

Gomery, T., Wong, S. E., Cohen, D., & Lacasse, J. R. (2011). Clinical social work and the biomedical complex. *Journal of Sociology and Social Welfare, 38*(4), 135–165.

Halsa, A. (2018). Trapped between madness and motherhood: Mothering alone. *Social Work in Mental Health, 16*(1), 46–61.

Hanson, R. F., & Lang, J. (2016). A critical look at trauma-informed care among agencies and systems serving maltreated youth and their families. *Child Maltreatment, 21*(2), 95–100.

Herman, J. L. (1992). *Trauma and recovery: The aftermath of violence – From domestic abuse to political terror*. New York: Basic Books.

Heward-Belle, S. (2016). The diverse fathering practices of men who perpetrate domestic violence. *Australian Social Work, 69*(3), 323–337.

Humphreys, C. (2011). Rebuilding together: Strengthening the mother-child bond in the aftermath of violence. *DVRCV Quarterly, 3*, 6–10.

Jackson, D., & Mannix, J. (2004). Giving voice to the burden of blame: A feminist study of mothers' experiences of mother blaming. *International Journal of Nursing Practice, 10*(4), 150–158.

Karban, K. (2017). Developing a health inequalities approach for mental health social work. *British Journal of Social Work, 47*(3), 885–992.

Kirk, S. A., & Kutchins, H. (1992). *The selling of DSM: The rhetoric of science in psychiatry*. New York: A. de Gruyter.

Kirmayer, L. J., Gone, J. P., & Moses, J. (2014). Rethinking historical trauma. *Transcultural Psychiatry, 51*(3), 299–319.

Lee, D. A. (2017). A person-centred political critique of current discourses in post-traumatic stress disorder and post-traumatic growth. *Psychotherapy and Politics International, 15*(2), e1411.

Macvarish, J., Lee, E., & Lowe, P. (2014). The 'first three years' movement and the infant brain: A review of critiques. *Sociology Compass, 8*(6), 792–804.

Moulding, N. (2017). Damned if you do, damned if you don't: Conflicted femininities in women's narratives of childhood emotional abuse. *Affilia, 32*(3), 308–326.

Muskett, C. (2014). Trauma-informed care in inpatient mental health settings: A review of the literature. *International Journal of Mental Health Nursing, 23*(1), 51–59.

Muzik, M., Bocknek, E. L., Broderick, A., Richardson, P., Rosenblum, K., Thelen, K. L., & Seng, J. S. (2013). Mother – Infant bonding impairment across the first 6 months postpartum: The primacy of psychopathology in women with childhood abuse and neglect histories. *Archives of Women's Mental Health, 16*(1), 29–38.

Naples, N. A. (2003). Deconstructing and locating survivor discourse: Dynamics of narrative, empowerment, and resistance for survivors of childhood sexual abuse. *Signs: Journal of Women in Culture and Society, 28*(4), 1151–1185.

Neal, P., Jackson, A., & McDermott, F. (2014). A review of the efficacy and effectiveness of cognitive-behaviour therapy and short-term psychodynamic therapy in the treatment of major depression: Implications for mental health social work practice. *Australian Social Work, 67*(2), 197–213.

Neukel, C., Bertsch, K., Fuchs, A., Zietlow, A., Reck, C., Moehler, E., Brunner, R. Bermpohl, F. & Herpertz, S. C. (2018). The maternal brain in women with a history of early-life maltreatment: An imagination-based fMRI study of conflictual versus pleasant interactions with children. *Journal of Psychiatry & Neuroscience, 43*(4), 273–282.

Neuro Resilience. (n.d.). *Mindfulness*. Retrieved from www.neuroresilience.net/mindfulness.

Pitts-Taylor, V. (2010). The plastic brain: Neoliberalism and the neuronal self. *Health, 14*(6), 635–652.

Raja, S., Hoersch, M., Rajagopalan, C. F., & Chang, P. (2014). Treating patients with traumatic life experiences: Providing trauma-informed care. *The Journal of the American Dental Association, 145*(3), 238–245.

Rimke, H., & Brock, D. (2012). The culture of therapy: Psychocentrism in everyday life. In D. Brock, R. Raby, & M. P. Thomas (Eds.), *Power and everyday practices* (pp. 182–202). Toronto: Nelson Education.

Rose, N., & Abi-Rached, J. M. (2013). *Neuro: The new brain sciences and the management of the mind*. Princeton: Princeton University Press.

Schechter, D. S., Moser, D. A., Reliford, A., McCaw, J. E., Coates, S. W., Turner, J. B., Serpa, S. R., & Willheim, E. (2015). Negative and distorted attributions towards child, self, and primary attachment figure among posttraumatically stressed mothers: What changes with Clinician Assisted Videofeedback Exposure Sessions (CAVES). *Child Psychiatry & Human Development, 46*(1), 10–20.

Stanford, S. (2010). 'Speaking back' to fear: Responding to the moral dilemmas of risk in social work practice. *British Journal of Social Work, 40*, 1065–1080.

Stark, E. A., Parsons, C. E., Van Hartevelt, T. J., Charquero-Ballester, M., McManners, H., Ehlers, A., Stein, A., & Kringelbach, M. L. (2015). Post-traumatic stress influences the brain even in the absence of symptoms: A systematic, quantitative meta-analysis of neuroimaging studies. *Neuroscience & Biobehavioral Reviews, 56*, 207–221.

Tseris, E. (2018). Social work and women's mental health: Does trauma theory provide a useful framework? *British Journal of Social Work, online first. Retrieved from* https://doi.org/10.1093/bjsw/bcy090

Vidal, F. (2009). Brainhood, anthropological figure of modernity. *History of the Human Sciences, 22*(1), 5–36.

Wastell, D., & White, S. (2012). Blinded by neuroscience: Social policy, the family and the infant brain. *Families, Relationships and Societies, 1*(3), 397–414.

Wendt, S., Buchanan, F., & Moulding, N. (2015). Mothering and domestic violence: Situating maternal protectiveness in gender. *Affilia, 30*(4), 533–545.

White, S. (2009). Fabled uncertainty in social work: A coda to Spafford et al. *Journal of Social Work, 9*(2), 222–235.

Zaleski, K. L, Johnson, D. K., & Klein, J. T. (2016). Grounding Judith Herman's trauma theory within interpersonal neuroscience and evidence-based practice modalities for trauma treatment. *Smith College Studies in Social Work, 86*(4), 377–393.

5 Dysfunctional and responsible

Women's accounts of therapeutic responses to gender-based violence

To complement the discussion in the previous two chapters relating to the contested meanings and implications of the trauma concept, this chapter turns its focus to reporting on qualitative interview research conducted with women regarding their negotiation of psychiatric and therapeutic discourses after violence. The experiential knowledges reported on in this chapter are valuable in contextualising the professional constructions of trauma presented in Chapters 3 and 4. The interview data demonstrate the pervasiveness of the influential trauma paradigm in constructing understandings of abuse and its effects. At the same time, the interviews demonstrate women's complex engagements with medicalised and therapeutic narratives of distress, including women's resistances to the totalising assumptions offered by the trauma paradigm. Following a brief discussion of the study's context and methodological approach, this chapter describes six major themes arising from the study: the complexities of medical diagnoses; conversations about abuse; the mixed benefits of therapy; therapy and self-management; therapy and isolation; and alternatives to therapy.

Narrative research processes

While mental health research is most often based on the assumption that objective, bias-free, and globally transferable knowledges can be established, critical perspectives on mental health – as discussed in Chapter 2 – have demonstrated the ways in which mental illness diagnoses are not neutral concepts but are instead shaped by socio-political, cultural, and historical contexts. Consequently, this study did not follow a positivist approach to knowledge-building intended to reach universal findings while ignoring the role of the researcher in interpreting and representing the voices of participants. Instead, it was informed by poststructural and feminist understandings of research. Rather than trying to eliminate bias, feminist research acknowledges the role of a researcher's subjective positioning within the research process (Ackerly & True, 2010) and recognises that research knowledge is political, context-bound, and embodied (Anastas, 2012). Notwithstanding the usefulness of quantitative methods in feminist research, qualitative approaches have been particularly valuable in achieving feminist aims as they produce data that allows for in-depth understandings, complexities, and contradictions to be presented (Denzin & Lincoln, 2003). Furthermore, qualitative approaches contribute towards knowledges that are context-bound, rather than aiming to generate data that is generalisable and transferable for the population at large (Malterud, 2000). Denzin and Lincoln (2003, p. 8) describe the iterative nature of qualitative analysis:

> There is no clear window into the inner life of an individual. Any gaze is always filtered through the lenses of language, gender, social class, race and ethnicity. Consequently, qualitative researchers deploy a wide range of interconnected interpretive methods.

A narrative research methodology was chosen for the study, due to its ability to value the perspectives of the participants and to record both their negotiation of and resistance to oppressive understandings of their identities (Langellier, 2001). Susan Chase (2011, p. 421) defines narrative as:

> [M]eaning making through the shaping or ordering of experience, a way of understanding one's own or others' actions, of organising events . . . or connecting and seeing the consequences of actions and events over time.

Chase (2011, p. 422) continues on to explore the functions of narratives in "identifying oppressive discourses and the ways in which narrators disrupt them". Thus, narrative inquiry is able to both name power operations and engage with participants' processes of resistance to the hegemonic narratives that seek to dominate understandings of their experiences and identities. Similarly, Stephens and Breheny (2013) argue that while narratives allow individuals to convey their personal experiences, they also reveal significant aspects relating to the structure of the social world. This approach fits well with the intentions of this study, as I did not want to situate the participants as merely passive recipients of medical and therapeutic discourses, thus painting a picture of immutable social forces and hopeless, victimised participants. Additionally, in line with the contributions of third-wave feminism outlined in Chapter 2, it was important to select a mode of inquiry that would leave space for the participants to express unfixed, multiple and fluid identities, and meaning-making processes (Butler, Ford, & Tregaskis, 2007). This study was particularly interested in critiquing the dominance of psychiatric and therapeutic narratives of women's distress, and searching for alternative knowledges of women's experiences. Narrative research is an invaluable tool in overturning traditional hierarchies of knowledge in mental health through its centralising of service user experiences, thus challenging biomedical orthodoxy and the silencing of service users' dissent (Sweeney, 2016). Narrative research is additionally helpful in its ability to draw together an analysis of structural disadvantage with an exploration of the emotional dimensions of inequality (Robinson, 2011).

Despite the benefits of narrative inquiry, however, there are a number of hazards or limitations that also need to be kept in mind, which are similar to the concerns have been raised by some feminists regarding the contemporary proliferation of "trauma" narratives and their individualising implications. As discussed in Chapter 3, while processes that create space for women to describe their previously invisibilised experiences of gendered oppression hold emancipatory potential, women's accounts of violence risk being read as individual tragedies that are insufficiently anchored in an analysis of the gendered power relations and other structural inequalities. In a similar vein, critical perspectives on narrative research have noted that the mere incorporation of first-person accounts into mental health research is insufficient in challenging mainstream psychiatric practices of assessment and diagnosis. In many cases, service user narratives are presented as an "empowering" research method in comparison to quantitative data collection, but in practice fail to transform conventional professional understandings. For example, they may rely on coding practices that evaluate participant quotations according to normative notions of "illness" and "dysfunction" and fail to engage with participants' critique of mental health services (Cohen, 2015). In addition, since participants do not construct their narratives within a social vacuum, narrative research may be limited in its capacity to produce new understandings of mental distress, as participants by necessity draw upon existing tropes and understandings to discuss their experiences (Moulding, 2016). In other words, due to the pervasiveness and influence of medical or therapeutic ideas and the lack of availability of other explanations, participants may use dominant discourses in order to explain their experiences, even if these understandings are personally disadvantageous or unsatisfactory. This creates complexities in the analytical process as oppressive constructions may appear to be freely chosen by participants, or otherwise, so pervasive that they are almost inevitable (Calder-Dawe & Gavey, 2017). Other concerns about narrative research include concerns about a lack of transparency about the role of the researcher in shaping the narratives that are constructed within the research process, and the notion that narratives are able to "speak for themselves", which is problematic for several reasons: it ignores how notions of the "self" change across contexts and time, it minimises the effects of social location on what people are able to observe, and it invisibilises differences and diversity among women (Hardesty & Gunn, 2017).

In focusing on participants' personal accounts of their lives, narrative inquiry is sometimes imbued with the unhelpful assumption that research participants negotiate the world as autonomous subjects, thus potentially being overly individualistic in its scope and minimising the effects of power relations on the lives of participants (Blumenreich, 2004). Additionally, narrative research often utilises extended direct quotations of participants' voices, which are implied to capture the "truth" of their experiences, leading to claims of objectivity despite the use of a qualitative methodology (Graham, 2005). Drawing out the complexities in participants' accounts rather than a singular narrative was therefore crucial in this study, and this was achieved through the utilisation of poststructural research principles. Poststructural narrative research attempts to produce a plurality of meanings, allowing for an array of tentative and multiple conclusions to be made (Adame & Knudson, 2007; Fraser, 2004). It is sceptical about binary positions and it contains the possibility of narrators who are at times "active" and at other times "passive" (Fullagar & O'Brien, 2013) – in other words, participants are not positioned in a simplistic and singular way in relation to hegemonic discourses, but rather are viewed as capable of taking up a multiplicity of positionings at various times. It aims not to settle upon the "truth" of participants' experiences, but to engage in participants' storying and re-storying processes in the construction of their identities (Riessman, 2008). A poststructural research framework searches for multiple realities, based on the premise that "there are many ways to be a woman, and these ways are fluid, dynamic, and shaped by the intersectionality of categories of difference" (Quiros & Berger, 2014, p. 153). This approach fits well with feminist research frameworks that aim to engage with the specificity of participants' accounts, in order to avoid coming to premature conclusions about the meanings of their experiences (Ackerly & True, 2010). It also enhances earlier feminist traditions, which have been criticised for only telling the stories of privileged women (hooks, 2000). This study endeavoured to critically engage with the "taken-for-granted" notion of trauma, with the aim of making sense of it as a socially constructed concept as it sought to interrogate trauma discourses in terms of how they constituted women and their experiences, and with what implications (Chambon, 1999). This meant that the analytical process attempted to avoid an assumption that trauma work has a singular meaning for participants, which has either universally positive or negative implications for mental health service users. Rather, the analysis explored the potential for the participants to develop multiple constructions of gender-based violence and trauma.

Interview processes

The deliberately broad criteria for participation in the study included women with experiences of abuse during their adolescence, within the context of a family relationship, currently aged over 18 years old. Recruitment strategies for the study included approaching non-government organisations, and advertising in the newsletters of not-for-profit human service agencies and community groups. In total, 18 women across a diverse range of age groups (mid-20s to mid-50s), with differing educational backgrounds, employment circumstances and income levels, and from a variety of locations including capital cities and regional areas in Australia participated in the study either in-person or through a telephone interview. Participants discussed a range of experiences of abuse including emotional, physical, and sexual abuse. However, a limitation of the study was that the majority of participants identified as having an Anglo-Celtic cultural background. Although not specified in the recruitment information, the participants relayed extensive experiences of medical and therapeutic interventions relating to multiple mental health diagnoses, including mood disorders, anxiety and PTSD, but participants did not discuss being diagnosed with any "psychotic" illnesses. There was an overrepresentation of participants who were themselves employed within the human service sector.

Participation was voluntary, and participants were advised of the option to withdraw from the study at any time with no adverse consequences. To ensure confidentiality, participants' names and other identifying criteria were kept confidential. Participants were interviewed using an in-depth, semi-structured interview approach. This approach used open-ended questions, in an attempt to generate detailed accounts of their experiences and perceptions (Engel & Schutt, 2009). Interview guides offered general topics to cover, but while some of the themes produced within the interviews were addressed directly by planned interview questions, others emerged more spontaneously. Additionally, the interview questions evolved over time to ask future participants to reflect on the emergent themes and issues. Core elements of narrative interviewing that were integrated into the study included an invitation to participants to discuss specific instances or memories from their lives, rather than relying solely on questions that asked participants to generalise about their experiences "as a whole" (Chase, 2011); the interviews were conversational and efforts were made to establish rapport and to demonstrate sensitivity (Fontana & Frey, 2003); time was spent sharing my emerging interpretations rather than treating participants as uninvolved in the analytical process (Kvale, 1996); and, where possible, I attempted to follow participants down their "trails of thought", which necessitated me to share power with participants, rather than exert complete control over the interview process (Riessman, 2008). This more iterative approach enabled me to be more open to the complexities within the participants' stories rather than being constrained by pre-defined topics or categories.

Ethical considerations and interview processes

A key concern when interviewing survivors of abuse is to avoid an interview process that may be harmful, a possibility that is heightened if participants are asked to recount their experiences repeatedly, or are asked intrusive questions (Walter & Rosen, 1997). With this in mind, participants were encouraged to disclose their experiences only to a level at which they felt comfortable. As the participants were over 18 years old, there was some distance from the adolescent period and the experiences that they were describing. The research adopted a relationship-based interview approach that aimed to position – as far as possible – the participants as "experts" relating to their own experiences and provide space for participants to shape the interview process (Butler et al., 2007). Furthermore, decision points were incorporated into the interview guide to ask participants at various points whether they would like to continue (Fontes, 2004). Also incorporated into the research approach was a discussion prior to the interviews about participants' current safety from violence and abuse, as well as their current levels of subjective wellbeing, with the aim of coming to a collaborative decision about whether to go ahead with the interview. Discussing these issues involved a delicate balance between addressing these questions and trying as far as possible to avoid paternalistic practices. Therefore, I tried to limit the use of mental health language, I tried to not influence too heavily women's decision-making processes regarding whether or not they could participate, and women were not excluded simply on the basis that they had a mental illness diagnosis. Debriefing occurred following the interviews, in which participants had the opportunity to outline aspects of the interview that they had found helpful and unhelpful, and were invited to discuss anything further if they wanted to. This process also included the option of linking participants to formal or informal supports, if needed, however this was not a necessary step for any of the participants.

Analytical processes

Interviews were transcribed verbatim from the audiotapes. Data analysis did not begin only once all the interviews were conducted, but rather, occurred throughout the process of interviewing, and informed and improved the quality of future interviews. It was important that the analytical process avoided overly prescriptive methods, in order to engage with the complexity of the data and to develop meaningful and nuanced findings. As described by Riessman (2008), narrative analysis typically involves the examination of "brief, bounded segment[s] of interview text" (Riessman, 2008, p. 61). However, efforts were made to avoid de-contextualising narratives from their location within the broader interview transcript, recognising that "much . . . meaning depends on where [a narrative] is situated in the conversation" (Emerson & Frosh, 2004). Furthermore, although qualitative inquiry is often interested in identifying themes present across interviews, I was also interested in instances in which participants "stood apart" from dominant perspectives and offered alternative understandings (Stanford, 2007).

The research question that guided the study was: *How did the participants negotiate psychiatric and therapeutic discourses when discussing the effects of abuse and violence?*, and the analytical process focused on the ways in which participants defined and positioned themselves in relation to medical and therapeutic discourses. To do this, I looked specifically for psychiatric and therapeutic narratives told by the participants, as well as alternative or "maverick" narratives (Stanford, 2007). I was interested in locating the subject positions taken up by the participants at different points in their interviews, investigating the multiple ways in which participants defined and positioned themselves in relation to medical, therapeutic, and other narratives (Blumenreich, 2004). The analysis engaged in the dual processes of both examining the effects of medical and therapeutic discourses on women who have experienced violence, while also being informed by a poststructural viewpoint that understood power as "circulating" rather than an oppressive force acting on passive individuals (Foucault, 1980). I was informed by Fullagar's (2009) approach to understanding women's use of antidepressant medications and her desire to avoid naming women's engagement with psy-discourses as "good" or "bad", aiming to develop a more complex analysis of the participants beyond the binary opposition of being either "victims" of psychiatric discourses or as executing a successful resistance to psychiatry (Fullagar & O'Brien, 2013). To achieve this, the analysis of the data involved a consideration of how the participants accepted, resisted, and negotiated psychiatric and therapeutic discourses. However, this process was balanced with a recognition of the gendered and social contexts affecting participants' capacity to mount a critique of psychiatric and therapeutic hegemony, and a consideration of how these contexts differed among the participants.

Following Riessman (2008, p. 11), I asked, "are there gaps and inconsistencies that might suggest preferred, alternative, or counter-narratives?" This question was particularly helpful in evaluating the perspectives of participants who had engaged in discourses outside of conventional psychiatric and therapeutic assumptions. Thus, poststructural narrative inquiry was able to examine participants' complex processes of drawing upon and resisting dominant medical and therapeutic discourses, as well as to identify competing narratives found within the interviews relating to the experience of gender-based violence and its effects. My involvement in the interviews is included in many of the excerpts below, in order to demonstrate the co-constructed nature of knowledge creation within the research process (Kvale & Brinkmann, 2009).

Complexities of medical diagnoses

Although it was not an inclusion criterion for the study, each participant had been labelled with at least one psychiatric diagnosis at some point either during or in the period following their adolescence. Mental health labelling processes had multiple effects on participants' lives, with benefits including "order" (the utility of diagnoses in the development of a cohesive understanding of their distress, which enabled their experiences to be rendered intelligible) and "legitimacy" (the utility of diagnoses in identifying the severity of the abuse that they experienced, and its ongoing effects). Consequently, several participants were relieved and appreciative regarding their psychiatric diagnoses. At the same time, however, diagnostic processes acted to produce reductionist and deficit-oriented understandings of women's identities. For example, a participant described the difficulties in engaging with mental health professionals because of the ways in which psychiatric discourses resulted in her identity being diluted into a set of problems, which was not always reflective of her lived experience:

Talking to professionals, I guess, can be harder. Psychiatrists can be harder because you feel – I feel like a hypochondriac sometimes because when you go see them, you're not always feeling bad. Do you know what I mean? So you feel stupid sometimes. (1)

Psychiatric discourses therefore constrained the potential for detailed and dynamic discussions about life after violence. Participants experienced dissonances between psychiatric language and their own, more contextualised and embodied understandings:

INTERVIEWER: *How did it feel to have that diagnosis [anxiety and depression]?*
PARTICIPANT: *Well, interesting you ask. I didn't like it. I don't like the term. When I look at what my anxiety is, I can see that it's basically fear of life. And the fear grows. And then that impacts on my experiences in the world. (2)*

A small number of participants openly critiqued biomedical understandings of their distress, arguing that the problems they were experiencing were clearly caused by abuse and violence. The psychiatric approach was seen as alleviating symptoms but not addressing causes:

I was angry, that the doctors you know, just prescribed me with a pill rather than saying, "ok, let's get to the cause of this, what happened, why did it happen, what made you feel this way?" It was just like, "oh, ok, well here's your pill, you know, see you later" – the problems just kind of get swept under the carpet so – I think it's more anger that I have to take this medication to make myself feel better, rather than, I don't know rather than the people out there who can kind of do something about the issues in the first place to prevent them from happening. (3)

For some participants, a diagnosis of Post-Traumatic Stress Disorder (PTSD) combined the legitimising benefits of medicalisation with a social analysis of the causes of their "symptoms". PTSD allowed for the joint advantage of both legitimising processes of psychiatric labels, as well as the social explanation for the emergence of distress:

INTERVIEWER: *And what are your thoughts about PTSD?*
PARTICIPANT: *Well that's all right because it gives me a reason for why things are the way they are. But I like to tell that I've got that term. Also that's what I've been labelled with. But it helps me to understand. (4)*

The PTSD diagnosis was useful for another participant in allowing her to receive a disability support pension, providing her with much-needed financial resources for a short period of time. This participant also felt that unlike other diagnoses, PTSD located the problem "outside" of her, within a context of abuse:

INTERVIEWER: *Did you appreciate the diagnosis then?*
PARTICIPANT: *I did . . . it's that claiming the label – it was really frightening to do, you know, what it says about being on a disability pension . . . for me to understand that people can look at everything that I say and see that, you know, the problem wasn't me, which is what me ending up in the mental health system said. That the problem was me, not anyone else . . . The problem is you, you know, the wiring in your brain or whatever. This actually said "no, hang on a minute, I'm just as good a person – no different to anyone else". I'm very sensitive. Maybe that made a difference to how things affected me. But it's all a result of the environment that I lived every single day of my in. So that way it was very helpful. (5)*

The participant was also buoyed by her belief that she was not fully defined by a psychiatric label, and that any classification assigned to her was merely a short-term description:

Well now I think labels are only useful insofar as like I have a motto that's "Claim It. Clean It Up and Throw It Away". If a label is useful for a while in reading all the research and information that people have come up with around it. . . . Then you can reach a point where you're free of it and that label doesn't apply. You can let it go. It's not who you are or anything. (5)

This belief in the flexibility of labels contrasted with another participant's less hopeful understanding that her diagnosis of Dissociative Identity Disorder was a "fixed" or immoveable component of her identity:

I wish I never had it but I do so I've got to live with it. (6)

In this way, the psychiatric label was experienced as an objective entity, wherein her identity was framed by fixed and defining characteristics. Neuroscientific discourses regarding the effect of trauma on the physical brain had a similar effect of "fixing" onto clients a "new identity" following trauma. The notion that neuroscience could be relevant to trauma recovery was highly appealing to many participants:

I do think that it's affected my memory, because I'm quite interested in the neuroscience and everything and I think it's really quite fascinating. As technology advances, they just understand so much more and I've just been to a couple of seminars recently at my kids' school, it's a psychologist, a developmental neuropsychologist, something like that. . . . So it's just something that's in the back of my mind at times, I'd really like to understand what happened to my brain. (7)

Brain-based discourses on trauma increased the capacity of labels to attach meaning to experience and enhanced deterministic assumptions made about the effect of childhood trauma on adult "functioning":

There was trauma early on, the way I understand it, it changes the way your brain's wired, and just even, if you're under a lot of stress, those teenage years, I was under a huge amount of stress, at the same time I was going through puberty, that's going to have an effect. Currently now, my diagnosis is anxiety and depression and just sort of knowing that is just because of what I went through. (8)

Neuroscience validated and confirmed the negative effects of abuse, acting as an authoritative discourse, through which a social explanation was made legitimate. Some participants sought out knowledge about the impact of traumatic experiences on the physical brain. Neuroscientific discourses added both legitimacy and certainty to their experiences of the relational effects of abuse:

Educating that young person about how trauma does impact on relationships and on the brain and that as well. So that they actually – because knowledge is power so at least you can – like if they know why they behave the way they do or whatever, that's helpful I think. (4)

Neuroscientific discourses therefore provided a pathway for the consequences of violence on women to be recognised; however, drawing upon them resulted in the detrimental effects of abuse being perceived first and foremost in terms of their effects on the brain.

Conversations about abuse

The secrecy of the abuse was a common issue raised, with the majority of the participants reporting that few people knew about the abuse that was happening to them during their adolescence. For some participants, mental health "symptoms" were the only avenues through which they were able to express their distress:

Probably that escalating problem that I had about that phobia was just about how I was expressing my distress about the abuse. Even though it was a bit extreme, it was a more valid way of expressing my problem rather than talking about it because I had no words. (7)

Within a context of secrecy, shame, and the difficulty of disclosure, participants described the need for mental health workers to be aware of the "signs" and "symptoms" indicating possible abuse and to end a reliance on the necessity for young people to explicitly disclose in order for an intervention relating to probable abuse to be put in place. For example, a participant argued that mental health symptoms in young people are indicators of abuse that professionals should be aware of, and that practitioners should remove the pressure to disclose from young women who are not ready:

Well if they're already in – like if they've already been say scooped up by the system, obviously they're expressing behaviours. I would say behaviours, no matter what they are, are always the symptoms and you need to know what questions to ask and what are the likely things that lead to those behaviours because they're always a cry for help. And if people – if the young people aren't saying to you outright, what's been done to them, you need to just accept – you need to know obviously something has happened. But the other thing is that you don't even need to know. Your first thing to do isn't to try and wheedle it out of them with words. You don't need to dig. It's not about that. . . . You're not triggering them back into stuff. They're choosing to bring it out, you know, what it literally was. Or they might never do that. (5)

Participants discussed the need for professionals to be informed about the prevalence of abuse and to use this knowledge to perceive abuse even when a young woman is not yet talking about it, and they were adamant regarding the need for professionals, and adults in general, to immediately and unreservedly believe young people when they disclose. However, when young people are unable to disclose, women suggested that workers should continue to consider the possibility that abuse has occurred. Sitting with the possibility that a young woman may not be able to tell the "whole story" about abuse initially (if ever) was described by women as a practice of "seeing beyond" spoken words, rather than "not believing" the young person:

PARTICIPANT: *Obviously with chronic absenteeism and coming to school with no lunch, bruises and all of those sorts of things, no one ever said anything, so I guess that would probably be one of the hardest things at my school, even though to be honest with you I did do a lot to kind of hide what was going on. I did make sure it looked like I was like everybody else. But I still think that that as teachers and educators and school counsellors, as experts in the field that they should have picked up a little bit more or being a little bit more mindful. Obviously I feel like, as a system, they should have done more, even though I was obviously doing my best to throw them off the scent – as the experts they should have been able to . . .*
INTERVIEWER: *Read between the lines?*
PARTICIPANT: *Yeah, exactly, and not just take my word for it – everything else, all the other indicators were ticked. (9)*

Some participants relayed the unhelpful aspects of direct questioning about abuse, stating that detailed investigations about abuse at the beginning of the therapeutic relationship could decrease the likelihood of disclosure:

I found it very invasive at first, I felt very, I don't know how to explain it, very caught off-guard if you like. And I didn't really know what to do, except pretend everything was OK. I guess maybe I thought I was going to get in trouble, or something. So I didn't want to get in trouble. Certain things had been identified by whichever teacher or my year advisor or whoever had sent me there and obviously that was the concern and that's what she went straight into and I just freaked out. I didn't want to get in trouble. (9)

Such concerns mirror a focus on safety as a key tenet of trauma-informed practices, which risks becoming lost in more recent attempts to develop screening tools relating to trauma, as outlined in Chapter 3. This participant went on to discuss how she experienced the questionnaire approach to assessment as reducing, rather than enhancing, professionals' capacity to hear stories of violence. Importantly, in many cases participants did want to be asked about abuse, and they wanted the behavioural and emotional indicators of abuse to be noticed and acted upon, even if they felt unsafe to explicitly disclose details. A participant spoke about her desire for a conversation about abuse to be possible in the future, despite her current inability to disclose that anything was wrong:

PARTICIPANT: *There was an occasion when a teacher did take me aside and try and speak with me and as I recall it being something like "you're often the happiest person but we notice that you're very down quite often" you know.*

And "do you want to talk about it?" And I remember just sort of saying "oh no, not really" and thinking: ask me again. Ask me again. But she didn't.

INTERVIEWER: *How did it feel to be asked how you are and do you want to talk?*

PARTICIPANT: *Look, I've always remembered that. Well it was fairly kind of, you know, I was sort of a "poetry writing" sensitive child. And so it's made me – I deal with people, I tend not to take the first answer, you know what I mean? I kind of think "yeah, look maybe someone does want to talk but they're not used to talking". You know what I mean? I wanted her to ask me more. I wanted to talk. But then I didn't know. I didn't have a story to sit there and go "blah, blah, blah".*

INTERVIEWER: *That's very interesting.*

PARTICIPANT: *I think it is – it's interesting in the sense that I don't think all young people are necessarily going to come in and give you the story. I mean, sensitive to other people that their first answer isn't necessarily the only one. (10)*

Another participant discussed the need for a slow, respectful approach to asking about abuse, in which young women are given time to feel that they will be supported in their disclosure:

PARTICIPANT: *Well I think you have to go very slowly for a start. Because it's too much – too quick is too much. You need that continual reinforcement and validation of "There's nothing wrong. This is normal. You are not the only person".*

INTERVIEWER: *And how would you have wanted to be asked? Would you have wanted someone to ask you just directly or what would have worked for you?*

PARTICIPANT: *I think somebody who has been specially trained in those areas will know the right questions to ask, without – you can't be straightforward. Did your father abuse you? Or did your grandfather abuse you? Because I'm telling you, the kids will just go "what are you insane, no way". . . . There has to be a way to be able to say it without coming straight out with it. . . . I just think there needs to be some specific timing in that area because you just can't come out and say "do you think you might have suffered sexual abuse?" or "do you think you might have been hurt?" (11)*

A further comment on the use of trauma "inventories" or standardised questioning tools about abuse noted the problem-saturated perspective offered by an investigative approach to the assessment of abuse and the overwhelmingly negative effects this had on her as a service user:

I've seen psychiatrists in the past ten years, and they always go into, have you had any abuse, and they go through the list, so they're always checking to see what this history is. It's long-winded, because there's a lot of history to go through, so you're usually pretty exhausted at the end of it. But, I know one time . . . after going through that experience, I was like "oh my goodness, I'm a mess. My life is a mess, I'm never going to get over it", that whole doomsday kind of feeling. Just because I'd gone through all of it, but it then left me with this "oh my goodness" I'm never going to get to the end of being ok. (8)

Therapy and mixed benefits

The terms "therapy" and "counselling" were used interchangeably in the interviews, to refer to formal talk-based interventions regarding emotional distress, in comparison to medication-based interventions, or non-professional supports, discussed later in this chapter. A large number of participants relayed the limitations of therapeutic approaches and frameworks in responding to their needs. They were offended by the lack of time taken by professionals to examine the individual aspects of their lived experience. In doing so, they demonstrated their own knowledge and meaning-making practices, which were ignored within a standardised intervention:

INTERVIEWER: *Can I ask about your opinions about therapy then, in terms of what it can and maybe can't achieve for people who have experienced abuse?*

PARTICIPANT: *I think that the therapeutic relationship has huge amounts of potential. I think that it's largely around "the who", probably over and above any theories on it. . . . I remember going to a psychologist and at a point I actually felt sorry for the guy . . . he tried to – I think probably a behavioural sort of approach, just a textbook, throw the theory at it, and very sort of artificial questions and in the end I felt so sorry for him. (12)*

For another, a technocratic professional encounter failed to honour the realities of her lived experience, especially her survivorship:

INTERVIEWER: *So could I just go back and ask if you have had a bad experience of therapy or counselling?*

PARTICIPANT: *Oh God I would walk out of there every time feeling like I was so profoundly flawed and so without the resources and such a hopeless case that I would never ever get anywhere. Like she was just – she had a fixed idea in her head about things. . . . And I was so angry. I said, "Wait a minute. I've been in this all these years. What are you talking about?" (13)*

A further understanding positioned an ideal therapeutic encounter as being informed by research but also heavily context-bound, tentative, and responsive to the individual. This participant expressed a desire for certainty, including drawing on brain-based discourses, but this occurred alongside a recognition of the limits of current knowledge and practices guidelines for trauma:

INTERVIEWER: *What sort of therapeutic work would have been helpful to sort of set you up as an adult in the best way possible?*

PARTICIPANT: *Well I think that they should be trauma-informed. And have an understanding of how trauma affects the brain and then how that in turn affects behaviour. And I think that they should also be aware that it should be ok for a person to sit in a room and not say anything. . . . I think everyone's just so busy trying to get you to follow their program or their list of things that should be done to make you better, that they lose sight of it's all very individual. (4)*

In spite of these substantial concerns, with few exceptions, participants situated therapy as an indispensable resource in managing the effects of violence, both during and in the aftermath of abuse. In fact, the majority of participants viewed therapy as the singularly most effective response to violence, rather than as one option among many valid strategies. One participant, for instance, believed that a complete immersion in therapy would result in her distress being entirely alleviated:

INTERVIEWER: *How important do you think counselling is to recovery?*
PARTICIPANT: *I think it's very important. . . . But also, you know, I think if I can stop work for 6 months and go to therapy every day I think I'd come out on top of the world. (1)*

Therapy occupied a privileged space, due to a widely held belief in its fundamental role after abuse:

INTERVIEWER: *What is your opinion about recovery from trauma?*
PARTICIPANT: *Probably, I think it would involve a lot of counselling. A lot of therapy to maybe, to deal with the situation, to cope with it. To get over it. I think it would just involve a lot of talking. (3)*

This view was held by the participant, despite the limitations of therapy that she had personally experienced:

It was really good for me to talk to someone like that. But at the end of the day, I still was suffering quite badly, like in terms of, I couldn't eat, I couldn't sleep, I felt like I couldn't function, so the talking, it was good, but it didn't help me function as a normal person. (3)

This perspective mirrored several participants' discussions of therapy as both a "commonsense" and highly valuable response to violence, even within a context of their own highly negative experiences of seeking professional help:

INTERVIEWER: *Even though you've had many bad experiences of counselling, you still think that counselling is very important?*
PARTICIPANT: *It is as long as you've got the right person . . . so maybe they need to hire more counsellors. I don't know. (6)*

Additionally, therapy was thought to be of immense help even within a context of highly supportive relationships outside of a therapeutic context, including friends and family who were open to discussing the effects of abuse and supporting the person through these experiences. For example, a participant described receiving very good support from a friend and her partner as a young woman attempting to understand her childhood experiences of sexual assault. However, she thought that she would have been benefited further through also having access to a professional to speak to about her experiences. She expressed her opinion that professional therapists are more adept at supporting people through difficulties than friends and family:

INTERVIEWER: *Can I ask, what is your opinion about the role of therapy in helping with the effects of abuse?*

PARTICIPANT: *I guess for anybody really, even if you have got people that you can talk to, you need people who can sort of direct your thinking and help you develop coping skills and understanding of things. Whereas people around you are probably too close, you need someone objective to help you deal with everything. (7)*

In this way, expert support was understood as having the capacity to impart certainty and objectivity, in contrast to the more fluid support offered by friends and family. Consequently, therapy occupied a privileged position as a normative and "common sense" response to violence. Conversations about the necessity of therapeutic interventions occurred even when therapy had been experienced as ineffective or detrimental. The limitations of therapy as a strategy to curtail the effects of violence were rendered invisible in these conversations, and other possible avenues and responses to abuse were minimised.

Another narrative thread within the participants' narratives was the construction of the emotional effects of abuse as immense, all-encompassing and escapable only through the therapeutic process. The majority of participants articulated the need to reduce and control their emotional distress, which was referred to using medical language such as "symptoms" and "recovery", as well as the term "trauma". Participants believed that professional support made "recovery" possible:

I realised I just wasn't recovering. I went and saw someone. (10)

Here, the participant positions herself as in need of professional expertise in order to help her to manage her limited capacities following abuse. The elimination of distress, or "recovery" was often positioned as the only viable or reasonable goal after violence. Participants framed their distress as unacceptable and as "fixable" through therapy. For example, a participant described the need to swiftly address distress with professional support:

I was just lucky I got help. But I think if you just let that escalate, if you didn't have help, it would be pretty horrible place to be and see how you're really depressed or mentally very unwell. (14)

Here, the discussion of getting "help" is imbued with notions of responsibility-taking. The participant constructs herself as a person in need of "fixing" and her distress following violence is situated as problematic. Her description of women who "just let [distress] escalate" demonstrates that women who do not participate in therapeutic processes in order to control their emotional pain after abuse risk the judgement of others. Women who engaged in therapy were viewed as taking an appropriate pathway towards recovering from the effects of abuse, through actively working on self-betterment:

> *I needed to work through a lot of issues and problems. I think the counselling helped me to build those strategies for myself and those coping mechanisms, so now that I have those coping mechanisms, it doesn't affect me as much as it did when I was 14 or when I was younger. (15)*

Therapy enabled participants to understand violence and its effects in particular ways, drawing attention to its psychological and personal effects. In defining the effects of violence, therapy drew attention to a "damaged" or "traumatised" inner self:

> *I found a really good psychologist. . . . I think by then I got enough of a picture that I don't know if I'd read about it or he had talked about it, complex post-traumatic stress disorder . . . it's to do with – maybe one or maybe more incidents of trauma that affect, you know, how you're operating in the world. But complex post-traumatic stress disorder is an ongoing, everyday trauma that affects your sense of yourself in the world. (5)*

In this way, therapy provided a language that enabled the participant to describe the aftermath of violence as being characterised by a personal psychological injury. This understanding of the "self" allowed her to experience validation regarding her distress, but it came at the cost of viewing herself as deficient and in need of expert assistance in order to gain a sense of competency and wellbeing. Indeed, the concept of "trauma" had a variety of consequences for participants. On the one hand, it enabled participants to articulate (sometimes for the first time) the injustices they had experienced:

> *It's just that fear that I could be killed, which is, that's probably the worst sort of trauma that a kid can sort of go through – just that fear of being murdered. (16)*
> *I have got a very serious case of post-traumatic stress syndrome, which has been cumulative over the years, starting with my childhood, and that's comprised of being physically and emotionally abused brutally. (17)*

However, the trauma discourse also had the effect of placing significant constraints on participants' capacity to view themselves as fully functioning adults with identities outside of the abuse they had experienced:

> *On reflection as an adult, I went and got some counselling, probably about 3 years ago. And the counsellor said to me, "Oh, you've had a very traumatic*

childhood". I said, "I didn't have a traumatic childhood" – and I'd normal-ised it so much for myself that I really didn't see the impact that violence had on me as a child, and then as an adult through life. . . . After I went through counselling [I] really sort of recognised the impact that the childhood trauma has had on me throughout my life. (16)

Here, the participant describes how the discourse of trauma introduced in the ther-apeutic interaction helped her to understand her life as being strongly impacted upon by her experiences of child abuse, however the discourse also resulted in a new-found perception of herself as vulnerable and "altered" by the violence. The concept of trauma privileged a focus on the emotional parts of the self, which were thought to be strongly affected by the violence. This focus had complicated conse-quences for participants, in that it both allowed for increased self-acceptance, as well as focusing participants' energy on the demanding task of continual manage-ment of internal states:

For a long time I would be really hopeful that everything was gone from my life and I didn't ever feel any difficult feelings again and would be happy. I think what I understand now is I may have intense big feelings on a regular basis for the rest of my life. But it's about accepting that. (5)

Thus, while participants experienced the trauma discourse as an effective means of validating their otherwise invisible experiences of abuse and its effects, this validation was entangled with understandings of individual pathology and per-sonal inadequacy:

I've been diagnosed with post-traumatic stress disorder. And I've been seeing a psychologist for the last probably two and a half years. I'm working and that but sometimes I find that hard to manage. But the majority of the time that's ok. (4)

Consequently, while the concept of trauma "gave voice" to participants' experi-ences, it remained heavily reliant on therapeutic constructs pertaining to individ-ual deficiencies when understanding and making meaning of violence. Although it named a contextual basis for participants' distress, the emphasis remained on internal and personal vulnerabilities, and the requirement to access "expert" pro-fessionals was viewed as essential.

Therapy and self-management

This chapter thus far has outlined the ways in which therapy constructed women as vulnerable and in need of expert assistance following abuse. In addition, understandings of the role of therapy that were described by participants simul-taneously positioned women as centrally responsible for adjusting to and manag-ing the effects of violence. As a result, therapy offered delimiting expectations regarding participants' capacities, while also expecting participants to engage in conscientious "help-seeking" behaviours. For example, participants spoke about not wanting to engage in therapy as a young person, but feeling as though they should have:

I think if the child – if the teenager can be – if the human being can be opened to it, then I think it's absolutely – it can be life changing. And if it's done well and it's done respectfully. And I don't know how you introduce it to a teenager who is resistant to it really. (13)

Another participant discussed the need to engage in therapy, even though she did not want to:

I was very shut off to counselling, I was very shut off to a lot of things, I'd just sort of wanted to . . . leave it alone. I suppose when I was going through a lot of traumatic things the only way for me to recover was just coping and learning how to cope. How to be able to deal with things, how to be able to make yourself happy, how to be able to get yourself out of a depressing situation at the time, if things are affecting you. (15)

In this way, therapy was constructed as an unpleasant experience, but as the action taken by a person who is taking responsibility. Even though the participant contextualised her distress as stemming from child sexual abuse, she was under pressure from herself and others to learn about effective self-management techniques in therapy to reduce the distress, and to then practise these regularly in order to achieve effective "symptom reduction". Discussions about therapy revealed the ways in which it provided "strategies" for coping with distress, which women were then expected to perfect through their own diligent exertion:

I've been diagnosed with PTSD and dissociative disorder. Recovery? The cognitive therapy I was doing was one they do for Vietnam vets. That's what I was trying to do, was retrain all that side of it. (1)

Here, the participant draws upon co-existing discourses of expert strategies, as well as the concept of individual effort. Conversely, another participant described an experience of therapy in which the notion of clients possessing few resources and being in need of expert guidance was avoided:

He was really positive, I remember him saying to me, things like, why are you such a really nice, respectful person? Where have you learnt that from? You know, "you've had an awful life, but yet you've come out and you're really polite and you're really genuine". (8)

This respectful and straightforward approach was experienced by the participant as extremely helpful. The therapist in this situation challenged both the "deficient client – expert therapist" discourse, and did not hold an expectation that she engage in strategies involving individual effort and self-management. The notion of individual effort had both affirming and disempowering implications for participants, in that it provided hope that overcoming the trauma of abuse was possible, but it also placed the majority of responsibility for trauma "recovery" onto individuals, who were expected to "cope" with life, regardless of injustice:

Trauma recovery? I guess my understanding for that would be is that there's light at the end of the tunnel. It's not going to always be darkness. There is a way out. There is a way to bust out, I guess, is the word I'm trying to look for. The hope that you can get your life back. It doesn't matter how many times you get knocked down, just get up and do it again. Eventually you will lead a normal life to a point. (6)

Here, the participant draws upon the optimistic metaphor of "light at the end of the tunnel" and she is energised by her belief in her personal resilience ("there is a way to bust out"). However, she is also burdened by the requirement to "just get up and do it again". There is also a sense in her narrative that her "recovery" will be partial and conditional ("you will lead a normal life to a point"). In this way, therapy's use of the self-management discourse operated in both energising and discouraging ways to produce women's understanding of their experiences. Nevertheless, a number of participants also challenged the discourse of individual effort. In fact, the notion of "resilience" itself was heavily contested by a number of participants, who situated resilience as a term that set up overly optimistic expectations regarding positive outcomes after violence, and that isolated the individual in their distress if they were not able to achieve these outcomes. Some participants were interested in re-defining resilience as survivorship on their own terms rather than as a normative pathway towards "symptom reduction":

INTERVIEWER: *What would be your understanding of resilience and do you think you are resilient?*
PARTICIPANT: *Do I think I'm resilient? Yes. I'm alive. . . . Anyone who survives anything like that, they're resilient. They're bloody resilient. (11)*

Thus, the participant defined herself as resilient outside the constraints of the restrictive self-management discourse. Another participant also defined resilience as being beyond individual capacities and effort:

And I think my understanding of resilience has changed a lot over time. I would have said resilience, once upon a time, was being able to be self-sufficient and not dependent on anybody and all that. Obviously, very well presented. Now I see resilience as having internal supports, you know, and knowing when you need support from outside and being able to get it for yourself. And having confidence that that support is going to be what you need and that you'll be able to make good use of it. (5)

Here, the notion of resilience as being an individual trait that a person possesses is challenged, demonstrating the limitations of the self-management model of recovery. Additionally, the participant drew a link between self-management and the attainment of socially appealing norms, showing that a focus on an all-sufficient self is only one way of understanding "recovery". She argued that while the pursuit of independence through therapy may result in a perception of resilience, this may not correlate with a person's experience of wellbeing, and the emphasis on the "self" risked undermining her external resources.

Another concern within participants' narratives about therapy was the fear that they could not successfully navigate their "ordinary lives" while being required to expend copious amounts of energy "working on" their emotional self:

But to exist today in a normal society, I have to work. I have to make money. I have to be able think without being on the verge of crying every five minutes. So when we try and get into it, it can be – it triggers all these emotions inside, and they have been buried for so long, it gets a bit hard for me to do normal things. To exist normally, like I've tried to do. (1)

In this way, the participant discussed the unreasonable expectations that were placed on her within a therapeutic context, and the unsustainable nature of therapy. Another spoke about the demanding process of therapy:

I think there are times when it's just too difficult. Because [therapy] does resurface all the emotions again and it – I just know a couple of friends – they've gotten to the point where they've started but it's opened up so many wounds. It's hard – it's that catch 22 but I also know that without it, there's no freedom from it – there's no closure or acceptance or whatever. (8)

Participants therefore expressed that therapy had complicated implications in their lives. While the notion of taking responsibility in order to develop successful "coping strategies" enabled some participants to experience themselves as successful and competent, it also contributed to other participants feeling as though they had failed in their attempts to "recover". Although an aspect of the "recovery" discourse involved participants talking to "experts" about their distress, the notion of self-management ultimately positioned the management of distress as being the responsibility of the individual, resulting in the invisibilisation of social and gendered contexts. As a result, participants placed the supposedly empowering concept of resilience under scrutiny.

Therapy and isolation

Mirroring influential humanistic notions of the importance of empathy within therapeutic work, when asked about the role that therapy played in their lives, the majority of participants spoke about the fundamental role that therapy played in providing validation and support:

INTERVIEWER: *What is your understanding of the place of therapy or counselling in helping people?*

PARTICIPANT: *Well I think when you're only inside your own head, that's not a safe place to be if you're trying to work things out and if you do get confused, which I think that was part of it, trying to understand what I call post-traumatic stress symptoms. You can't deal with them on your own. So I think the counselling was really important. And I think talking about it as an adult, when I had had such a long period of not ever talking about it, which was my choice, gave some concreteness to what that experience was. It kind of gives some acknowledgement without overplaying it and becoming morbidly concerned about the fact that that happened as a child, it gives some relevance to that the fact that it wasn't in my mind, it actually did happen, if that makes sense. (14)*

In addition to the need for empathy and validation, this participant described a strong desire to reduce her isolation, and a number of other participants described similarly intense experiences of isolation, and their efforts to address this isolation by seeking therapy. Importantly, therapy was often only able to address the need for connection in peripheral ways. For one participant, therapy opened up a possibility to feel less alone and to understand others' experiences. Yet while the therapeutic relationship was extremely important for the participant, it reduced but did not resolve her isolation:

INTERVIEWER: *Could I ask what is your opinion about the role of therapy in helping people who have experienced abuse? How important is it?*

PARTICIPANT: *I think it's incredibly important. I don't know how you get out of this mess on your own. And it's one of the reasons we end up in the mess that we're in is because of the aloneness and the way that society does, you know, white western society, we do end up – so many of us end up separated and with a sense of aloneness and that it's just us. And it's therapy that introduces us to the possibility that it's not us personally, that these are experiences that have happened to lots of other people. (5)*

Here, the participant described the micro-context of isolation created through her abuse experiences. However, she also discussed a much broader context to her "aloneness", and the resultant effects on the capacity to experience community and connection, culminating in extreme separation. Within this context, therapy offered a potentially invaluable awareness of "lots of other people". Nevertheless, although some participants described their conversations in therapy as enabling them to understand themselves in relation to other survivors of child abuse, due to the constraints of therapy, this realisation was only able to occur on an intellectual level. Another participant spoke about the lack of opportunities for talking about the consequences that violence had had on her life, outside of a therapeutic context. She did not believe that her friends would be capable of providing support relating to her experiences:

You can't talk to your friends all the time about it because everybody's life is hard. You can't burden your friends. You don't know what goes on in their life. And their life is hard. Everybody's life is hard. So I don't talk to my friends that way because I don't want to burden them. (1)

In this situation, the availability of therapy arguably contributed to the participant's ongoing isolation. She did not believe that it was appropriate to seek her friends' support, worrying about the impact that her needs would have on them. The only support that she felt entitled to receive was within the context of a professional relationship. By setting up a binary opposition between personal and professional relationships, where abuse is only spoken of within professional relationships, the inability to connect with other women was reinforced. Another participant suggested that therapists could transform their practice from an individualised treatment approach to take on the role of connecting young people who had experiences of violence in common:

INTERVIEWER: *I just wanted to ask about if you think about reflecting on your experiences, what information would have been helpful to hear during your adolescence or what message?*

PARTICIPANT: *I think had I been connected to maybe other people that had been in a similar circumstance, so I was very on my own. And I think that could have helped. I think the fact that I couldn't really talk to my peers at school. Because you can't bring that up in conversation. But maybe having had a connection through a counsellor where I met other people might have made a difference to maybe not being so isolated on my own. (14)*

Participants thus destabilised an idealised understanding of therapy as being unproblematically supportive for women following violence. In fact, the separateness of therapy from the rest of their lives and its disconnection from other women at times may have heightened rather than alleviated their sense of isolation.

Alternatives to therapy

Despite therapy being understood as an indispensable course of action after violence by the majority of participants, there were alternative modes of relational support also identified within the interviews. For example, several participants spoke about the impact of abuse on their development of intimate partner relationships, in particular, the difficulties they experienced negotiating consent, understanding boundaries and exercising assertiveness:

No-one ever sat me down and said "What's the point of a relationship? How do you set healthy boundaries? How do you resolve conflict?" . . . No-one ever told me that I could choose when and where and how I wanted to [negotiate a sexual relationship]. (18)

For some participants, therapy was viewed as a fundamental pathway in enabling shifting understandings of relationships and moving towards feeling safe and connected. In the example below, the therapist encouraged the participant to view her needs in a relationship as valid, and articulated a relationship as a two-way process in which her partner might be involved in support and kindness regarding the experiences of fear and shame:

INTERVIEWER: *Can I ask about your – what are your opinions about therapy then, in terms of what it can and maybe can't achieve for people who have experienced abuse?*

PARTICIPANT: *I guess [the counsellor communicated] that anything that I'm feeling is valid. . . . And to say, "You don't have to run, when there's hard feelings there. You can find a partner who is safe enough to work things through with. You deserve that". And just being very clear that you didn't deserve anything that happened to you. There was nothing that you did that made it happen. (12)*

However, therapy was not the only avenue open to participants in moving towards the development of relational safety, and there were other significant relationships named by participants as helping them to learn about respect and empathy:

I was very lucky to have a grandmother who was a model of – although she didn't know what was going on, and she lived interstate and we had limited contact with her, she was a model for me – a role model for me in how to have intimate relationships and she and my grandfather had a beautiful relationship. And I think it was only because of seeing that, and knowing her intimately, that I was able to have intimate relationships. And that I met my husband very, very young and he is just an extraordinarily beautiful man who has been the saving of me in many ways. Very gentle and loving and accepting. I learnt from him a lot too. (13)

This perspective contrasts with other views that discussed the need for women to engage in therapy after abuse in order to learn about trust and boundaries in readying themselves for a future relationship.

I guess you need to change the way you think and maybe then you will attract the right kind of [man] you want. (6)

The construction of participants as lacking skills and knowledge as a result of their experiences situated the problem within the women themselves, and is reflective of some of the judgemental and blaming ideas about women's relational dysfunctions that are embedded within the Borderline Personality Disorder (BPD) diagnosis.

Within the interviews, participants were asked about their opinions regarding feminism and whether they believed that a feminist analysis was relevant in helping them to understand their experiences of violence. The majority of participants did not identify with a feminist identity and did not believe that feminism was a relevant framework for understanding abuse against young women, or they understood feminism as an abstract concept, and they expressed uncertainty about its relevance. In contrast to this ambivalent position, a few participants were strongly opposed to an analysis of violence that utilised a gender analysis, and it was at times difficult for women who were opposed to a feminist analysis to hold men accountable for their violence. Nevertheless, a small number of participants did identify as feminists and understood their experiences of abuse as being constituted by masculine privilege:

> *I am a very passionate feminist, so I do take part in as many things as I can, including protests. . . . I think, I think it helps to be able to kind of bring issues forward, make them more public, because I know that there's such a silence around the things that women go through. . . . I think it's important to get out there, publicly, and share stories with other women too. (3)*

Although the participant had participated in mainstream therapy and felt it was important for individual women to gain mastery over their trauma "symptoms", she eagerly discussed the need for political action and social change, and she felt proud about her involvement in feminist activities. She discussed the benefits of support from feminist allies in the aftermath of violence, above and beyond the benefits of therapy:

> *I think a lot of the times professional people can come across as very cold and clinical, and I don't think that helps at all. Like, I would prefer to talk to a feminist! (3)*

In a similar vein, another participant discussed how the legal justice that she was able to access was essential in the aftermath of sexual abuse. Not only did the legal process validate her personal experience, it also connected her to a broader context of other women with similar experiences and this inspired her to become involved in feminist politics within her rural community:

> *I think really for me, I think that the big thing was that because I was able to go to the courts, and he had his justice. . . . I am passionate about what I've been through and where I've come myself at this point. . . . So I suppose with that, because I've gone through that part of it, it's helped me to be able to be more open and talk about it with others. . . . I've just come to this point in time that I actually want to be more of an activist about this. (15)*

Although the participant discussed therapeutic "gains", the combination of feminist involvement and legal rights enabled her to move beyond these "therapeutic" gains, helping her to take on a new role in her community, feeling capable of being an advocate for others. In another arena beyond therapy, only a few participants were able to connect to a career pathway that was genuinely meaningful for them and that enabled them to experience a sense of competency. In fact, several participants experienced low workforce participation and poverty. For those women with stable and meaningful jobs, however, their career represented a fundamental component of their wellbeing. For example, one participant experienced her career as highly motivating and challenging.

At 33, I took on the [role of] CEO of this organisation. . . . All things being equal, I feel like I've come through the other side without it being heavily damaged in a way. I know it's with me [the sexual abuse]. It's not something that you just put away and – I kind of embrace it now that that's just part of who I am. I do what I do. I think it affects the fact that I am so determined, focused and try to do what I do for the benefit of other people. (14)

A career path enabled her to reconceptualise the possible effects of the abuse as strengths, rather than as symptoms in need of elimination. For another participant, work was not fulfilling in and of itself, but it did provide a sense of purpose and routine, which was valued:

INTERVIEWER: *And how important is work for you?*
PARTICIPANT: *Very. It's what keeps me going. It may not be the job that I love or expected to be in but I can do it and it keeps me going. (1)*

In this way, employment and a career pathway were not simply possible for women after they had "worked through" the "symptoms" of abuse; rather, they were fundamental to assisting women to either positively utilise or manage the effects of violence. Consequently, work not only provided what the therapeutic discourse claimed to provide – a respite from symptoms – but, at times, it did so more successfully. One participant's work as an artist was incredibly important to her as it allowed her to "give voice" to her survivorship that was not possible in any other context:

So it's a self-portrait that I'm doing [currently]. And really that whole experience I went through when I was a teenager I guess, is really the reason that that's a big part of why I'm doing the portrait. Just to signify that it's over and I survived and so that's really what art means to me. It's just a way of expressing myself really. (7)

The participant's artistic work differed from a therapeutic approach of focusing in on vulnerabilities in order to gain mastery over them; at the same time, her discussion extended beyond simplistic notions of resilience. By describing her experiences of abuse as meaningful, but not central in framing her current under-standings of "self", the participant problematised an essentialising view about the central role of abuse in identity-formation, while at the same time rejecting a linear notion of trauma recovery.

Implications and reflections

This chapter has demonstrated the complexities within the participants' engage-ment with dominant medicalised and therapeutic discourses in the aftermath of violence. Despite the participants' discomfort regarding mental health labels, finding ways to effectively resist psychiatric practices was a complicated process due to the mixed benefits afforded by diagnoses – in particular, the double-edged implications of the PTSD diagnosis. The trauma discourse constructed a coherent and validating narrative of distress, but its emphasis on symptom management within individuals usually precluded a fuller analysis of the gendered power rela-tions underpinning violence against young women. Neuroscientific discourses aided the problem-saturated, deterministic understanding of participants' lives provided by psychiatric labels, through promoting the notion of fixed, organically based changes occurring to traumatised women. At the same time, neuroscience was drawn upon by women attempting to legitimate a social explanation of their "symptoms", however this occurred through prioritising the role of the physical brain in the development of adverse outcomes.

A majority of the participants viewed therapeutic interventions as vital both during and in the aftermath of abuse. However, despite the privileging of therapy within the study's narratives, participants' positioning in relation to therapeutic interventions was often vexed and problematic. Consequently, while a "therapy as indispensable" discourse was articulated by several the participants, the notion that therapy is a centrally important response to violence and its effects was also problematised through their discussion of its mixed implications. The analysis of women's narratives found that therapeutic interventions rendered them as "dam-aged" human beings, while at the same time charging them with the responsibil-ity to engage in relentless self-monitoring and self-development. Thus, therapy placed women in a "double bind" by positioning them as being both in need of expert assistance *and* as responsible for managing the effects of abuse. Never-theless, participants were often reluctant to question the centrality of therapy as a response to violence and abuse. The participants were most highly critical of standardised interventions, in which the importance of providing safety and rec-ognising diversity were ignored or minimised. This is a particularly important finding in view of the increasingly standardised approach embedded within more recent iterations of trauma-informed practices.

Participation in therapy often provided a source of support and empathy, which participants frequently experienced as meaningful, but the limitations of the thera-peutic relationship contributed to ongoing experiences of isolation and despair. Trauma-informed guidelines usually include the notion of "collaboration" between workers and service users, but the interviews reveal the complexities within this aspiration, as participants discussed the power of therapists to impose frameworks of meaning, including notions of a coherent trauma trajectory, onto participants' experiences. Further, when notions of trauma were combined with neuroscience discourses, they were granted the status of objective knowledge. As a result, workers maintained control within the therapeutic interactions, reflecting Proctor's (2008) concerns about discourses of collaboration and their propensity to invite complacency by drawing on notions of partnership, while concealing the ongoing existence of a hierarchical relationship.

Deficit-focused and essentialising discourses about "traumatised" women emphasise internal pathology, leading to assumptions about the expected negative psychological outcomes that occur in women who have lived through violence and abuse. In contrast, this chapter has presented data suggesting that following abuse women do not necessarily enter a downward spiral of distress and pathology. While some participants experienced the effects of violence as ongoing and significant, for others, the experience of childhood abuse had more peripheral effects on their adult life. This finding problematises overly simplistic causal dynamics that are present within some understandings of trauma, and mirrors Briere and Jordan's argument that the complex effects of child abuse on adult "symptomotology" means that "it may be overly simplistic to refer to the effects of childhood abuse and neglect, per se" (Briere & Jordan, 2009, p. 383). Crucially, however, several participants reported significant, ongoing harm and a range of negative effects. Therefore, the participants were not affected in a uniformly predictable fashion, with some women finding ways to resist prescriptive understandings and meanings within the dominant psychological narrative of dysfunction following violence, while at the same time speaking back to neoliberal values relating to personal responsibility in the absence of adequate resources. Participants argued that resilience was not a "given", that it was often based on social resources rather than on internal strengths, and that a capacity to depend on others was important. They also noted that normative understandings of "resilience", which define resilience merely as individual perseverance, can at times lead to social isolation, or reduce a person's ability to access available support and resources. This finding reflects other critical research into resilience, which has highlighted the contested nature of resilience, and the need to attend to its varying meanings and implications (Ungar, 2011). In contrast to the idea that resilience is an individual trait, women's social contexts and resources mediated the processes that had occurred in participants' lives between their adolescence and the time of the interview, and not all women had access to the resources necessary for the development of normative markers of resilience, for example, a meaningful career or nurturing personal relationships.

As in all qualitative studies, the purpose of this research study has not been to produce findings of a highly generalisable nature, but rather, to engage with in-depth and nuanced accounts of women's experiences, which are concealed within quantitative research processes. The women who participated in the study reported extensive medical and/or therapeutic involvement in response to their experiences of gender-based violence and the study revealed the problematic and limited nature of many of these responses. Consequently, an important direction for future research is the intentional exploration of alternative approaches to supporting women who have experienced violence, as a means of disrupting the "common-sense" status that is currently afforded to medical and therapeutic responses. Another significant area that was not able to be examined in this study is a consideration of how the intersections of gender and race impact upon women's experiences and negotiation of dominant discourses of abuse and its effects. Finally, recent work on the use of service user narratives in academic research has highlighted the urgent need to work towards practices of inclusivity and equal partnership between researchers and service users within research processes (Russo & Sweeney, 2016). This goal represents a significant challenge for research practices in the area of critical mental health, particularly as social sciences research increasingly draws upon aspirational notions of "participation" and "co-production", while obscuring the ongoing power differentials that continue to exist between researchers and participants (Russo & Beresford, 2015).

Conclusion to the chapter

Many people do attend therapy hoping to feel better, and it is, of course, problematic to withhold potentially helpful strategies for alleviating women's distress on the basis that they do not address structural causes (Rosenthal, Reinhardt, & Birrell, 2016). Taking steps to alleviate individual emotional suffering and engaging in a sociological critique of the limitations therapy do not need to be mutually exclusive processes (Fook, 2016). Nevertheless, there are pitfalls involved in overstating the benefits of therapy and overlooking its inability to engage with the gendered causes of women's distress. Such hazards include directing a disproportionate level of resources to therapy as a solution to violence, at the expense of more systemic responses; placing pressure on women to continue to participate in therapy, regardless of its benefits; and situating the problem of disappointing therapeutic outcomes within individual women. The women's perspectives reported on in this chapter shed light on the fraught pathway offered by therapeutic responses to gender-based violence, as well as the mixed consequences of utilising trauma discourses to make sense of their experiences. This qualitative research work sets the scene for the next chapter, which provides some tentative ideas on how the challenges that have been raised so far in this book relating to the trauma concept might be effectively addressed. Chapter 6 discusses strategies relating to how the contested trauma paradigm might be strategically negotiated in order to achieve feminist and social justice aims within mental health settings and beyond, while acknowledging the pressing need for social actions taken outside of mental health services in the movement to end violence against women.

References

Ackerly, B., & True, J. (2010). *Doing feminist research in political and social science.* London: Palgrave Macmillan.

Adame, A. L., & Knudson, R. M. (2007). Beyond the counter-narrative: Exploring alternative narratives of recovery from the psychiatric survivor movement. *Narrative Inquiry, 17*(2), 157–178.

Anastas, J. W. (2012). From scientism to science: How contemporary epistemology can inform practice research. *Clinical Social Work Journal, 40*(2), 157–165.

Blumenreich, M. (2004). Avoiding the pitfalls of 'conventional' narrative research: Using poststructural theory to guide the creation of narratives of children with HIV. *Qualitative Research, 4*(1), 77–90.

Briere, J., & Jordan, C. E. (2009). Childhood maltreatment, intervening variables, and adult psychological difficulties in women: An overview. *Trauma, Violence and Abuse, 10*(4), 375–388.

Butler, A., Ford, D., & Tregaskis, C. (2007). Who do we think we are? Self and reflexivity in social work practice. *Qualitative Social Work, 6*(3), 281–299.

Calder-Dawe, O., & Gavey, N. (2017). Feminism, Foucault, and Freire: A dynamic approach to sociocultural research. *Qualitative Psychology, online first*. Retrieved from http://dx.doi.org/10.1037/qup0000106.

Chambon, A. S. (1999). Foucault's approach: Making the familiar visible. In A. S. Chambon, A. Irving, & L. Epstein (Eds.), *Reading Foucault for social work* (pp. 51–81). New York: Columbia University Press.

Chase, S. E. (2011). Narrative inquiry: Still a field in the making. In N. K. Denzin & Y. S. Lincoln (Eds.), *The Sage handbook of qualitative research* (pp. 421–434). Los Angeles: Sage.

Cohen, B. M. Z. (2015). *Mental health user narratives*. Houndmills: Palgrave Macmillan.

Denzin, N. K., & Lincoln, Y. S. (2003). Preface. In N. K. Denzin & Y. S. Lincoln (Eds.), *Collecting and interpreting qualitative materials* (2nd ed., pp. ix–xiii). Thousand Oaks: Sage.

Emerson, P., & Frosh, S. (2004). *Critical narrative analysis in psychology*. New York: Palgrave Macmillan.

Engel, R. J., & Schutt, R. K. (2009). *The practice of research in social work*. Los Angeles: Sage.

Fontana, A., & Frey, J. H. (2003). The Interview: From structured questions to negotiated text. In N. K. Denzin & Y. S. Lincoln (Eds.), *Collecting and interpreting qualitative materials* (2nd ed., pp. 61–106). Thousand Oaks: Sage.

Fontes, L. A. (2004). Ethics in violence against women research: The sensitive, the dangerous, and the overlooked. *Ethics and Behaviour, 14*(2), 141–174.

Fook, J. (2016). *Social work: A critical approach to practice*. London: Sage.

Foucault, M. (1980). *Power/knowledge*. New York: Harvester Wheatsheaf.

Fraser, H. (2004). Doing narrative research: Analysing personal stories line by line. *Qualitative Social Work, 3*(2), 179–201.

Fullagar, S. (2009). Negotiating the neurochemical self: Anti-depressant consumption in women's recovery from depression. *Health: An Interdisciplinary Journal for the Social Study of Health, Illness and Medicine, 13*(3), 389–406.

Fullagar, S., & O'Brien, W. (2013). Problematising the neurochemical subject of anti-depressant treatment: The limits of biomedical responses to women's emotional distress. *Health: An Interdisciplinary Journal for the Social Study of Health, Illness and Medicine, 17*(1), 57–74.

Graham, L. G. (2005). *Discourse analysis and the critical use of Foucault*. Paper presented at the Australian Association for Research in Education, Sydney. Retrieved from https://eprints.qut.edu.au/2689/1/2689.pdf.

Hardesty, M., & Gunn, A. J. (2017). Survival sex and trafficked women: The politics of re-presenting and speaking about others in anti-oppressive qualitative research. *Qualitative Social Work, online first*. Retrieved from https://doi.org/10.1177/1473325017746481.

hooks, b. (2000). *Feminism is for everybody*. Cambridge: South End Press.

Kvale, S. (1996). *Interviews: An introduction to qualitative research interviewing*. California: Sage.

Kvale, S., & Brinkmann, S. (2009). *InterViews: Learning the craft of qualitative research interviewing*. Thousand Oaks: Sage.

Langellier, K. M. (2001). Personal narrative. In M. Jolly (Ed.), *Encyclopedia of life writing: Autobiographical and biographical forms* (Vol. 2). London: Fitzroy Dearborn.

Malterud, K. (2000). Qualitative research: Standards, challenges, and guidelines. *Lancet, 358*, 483–488.

Moulding, N. (2016). Gendered intersubjectivities in narratives of recovery from an eating disorder. *Affilia, 31*(1), 70–83.

Proctor, G. (2008). CBT: The obscuring of power in the name of science. *European Journal of Psychotherapy and Counselling, 10*(3), 231–245.

Quiros, L., & Berger, R. (2014). Responding to the sociopolitical complexity of trauma: An integration of theory and practice. *Journal of Loss and Trauma, 20*(2), 149–159.

Riessman, C. K. (2008). *Narrative methods for the human sciences*. Los Angeles: Sage.

Robinson, C. (2011). *Beside one's self: Homelessness felt and lived*. Syracuse: Syacuse University Press.

Rosenthal, M. N., Reinhardt, K. M., & Birrell, P. J. (2016). Guest editorial: Deconstructing disorder: An ordered reaction to a disordered environment. *Journal of Trauma & Dissociation, 17*(2), 131–137.

Russo, J., & Beresford, P. (2015). Between exclusion and colonisation: Seeking a place for mad people's knowledge in academia. *Disability and Society, 30*(1), 153–157.

Russo, J., & Sweeney, A. (Eds.). (2016). *Searching for a rose garden: Challenging psychiatry, fostering mad studies*. United Kingdom: PCCS Books.

Stanford, S. (2007). *The operations of risk: The meaning, emotion & morality of risk identities in social work practice*. PhD, University of Tasmania. Retrieved from https://eprints.utas.edu.au/7688/.

Stephens, C., & Breheny, M. (2013). Narrative analysis in psychological research: An integrated approach to interpreting stories. *Qualitative Research in Psychology, 10*(1), 14–27.

Sweeney, A. (2016). Why mad studies needs survivor research and survivor research needs mad studies. *Intersectionalities, 5*(3), 36–61.

Ungar, M. (2011). The social ecology of resilience: Addressing contextual and cultural ambiguity of a nascent construct. *American Journal of Orthopsychiatry, 81*(1), 1–17.

Walter, G., & Rosen, A. (1997). Psychiatric stigma and the role of the psychiatrist. *Australasian Psychiatry, 5*(2), 72–74.

6   De-therapising trauma

Negotiating the contested trauma concept

Drawing on both critical literature and empirical data, this book has identified a number of challenges relating to the trauma paradigm's capacity to transform mental health systems into contexts where social justice for women who have experienced violence is possible. Although labelling women as "traumatised" is widely understood to provide an alternative and more empowering response than the dehumanising effects of mainstream psychiatric labels, it often gives rise to double-edged implications. The trauma concept can assist in providing a means through which women's emotional distress can be understood and validated, thus justifying the need for resources and support, but this acknowledgement comes at a cost. Frequently, the resources that are harnessed as a result of a label of "trauma" are limited to mental health and therapeutic services that are unable or unwilling to address socio-environmental factors or gendered power inequalities. Therefore, trauma discourses should not be viewed as inherently benevolent and effective in supporting the progression of women's rights; at the same time, they are not entirely problematic. The trauma paradigm provides an imperfect avenue through which women's often invisible experiences of violence can become intelligible and be elevated to the status of legitimate knowledge.

This final chapter attends to the challenging question of how trauma discourses might be effectively negotiated in order to achieve social justice outcomes for women. This exploration draws upon the work of scholars who have argued that a stand-alone critique of psychiatric discourses does not recognise the full effects that psychiatric labels exert upon people's lives (for example, Rose, 1999). Although the trauma lens is insufficient in fully achieving feminist aims in mental health settings and, in fact, is sometimes completely at odds with these aims, this chapter examines the ways in which it may be used strategically to create a counter-discourse within mental health environments that are otherwise saturated in biomedical constructions of women's distress.

Towards a critical analysis of trauma

This book has contributed to contemporary debates about trauma by arguing that while the contemporary trauma paradigm relating to gender-based violence may have a strong basis in feminist activism, its present-day broad usage means that there is no single paradigm of trauma or trauma-informed practices; rather the trauma concept has been utilised for diverse purposes, resulting in a variety of implications for women who have experienced violence, alongside other people whose interactions with the mental health system are informed by the trauma paradigm.

Although there are some indications that mainstream psychiatric discourse is becoming more tenuous, with some of its most outspoken critics coming from within the profession of psychiatry itself, it is unlikely that psychiatric discourses will be replaced in the near future. Instead, both people with feminist values entering the human service professions and women who become mental health service users are faced with the dilemma of how to negotiate the ongoing dominance of psychiatric constructions of human experience. Trauma-informed practices perform an obvious mediating function, allowing for more contextualised and gender-informed understandings of women's distress. However, versions of trauma that have been stripped of their political edge risk simply reinstating conventional understandings of women's mental distress, by acknowledging and yet ultimately covering over experiences of violence, focusing on symptoms, and imposing pre-determined meanings onto women's experiences. A commitment to feminist perspectives and critical mental health theory can be used to counter the contemporary tendency towards symptom-focused versions of trauma, and to ensure that trauma is not simply used as a de-facto mental illness categorisation, but retains its politicised capacities. In considering the various possible implications of trauma discourses, it is helpful to engage in a critical interrogation of the assumptions and power relations that underpin differing constructions of trauma. The following questions may act as a starting point when analysing constructions of trauma or trauma-informed practices:

1　Whose voices are being heard?

Are they professional, experiential, or both? If experiential narratives are present, are they being used to merely bolster professional models, or are they used to challenge the assumptions of mainstream mental health service provision? What theoretical frameworks are being used to contextualise service user knowledges? When research data is being used as evidence, what epistemological approach is being used – is it based upon notions of objective distancing from participants, with "experts" who are engaged in measurements or assessments? How much space is being given to the voices and perspectives of those who are being labelled as "traumatised"? How much certainty is being placed upon the understanding or model of trauma that is being put forward – is room being made for multiple perspectives and complex, non-linear narratives? Is a hierarchy of knowledges being established, with certain understandings being elevated above others (for example, diagnostic and neuroscientific discourses)?

2　Is professional power being extended or subverted?

Are there ways in which human service professionals may benefit from this version of trauma, for example, through expanded job opportunities and new diagnoses? Are simple assertions being made about the need for "more" mental health services to be established, and if so, whose interests do these statements serve? Is there a recognition that if improvements were to be made to women's social positioning, rights and safety, that fewer mental health services would be required? Is space being made to question the limitations of both medical *and* therapeutic responses to gender-based violence? Are the responses that are being offered viewed as optional, or as essential and universally relevant? Are alternatives to conventional medical and therapeutic responses being offered? Is consciousness-raising part of what is being offered?

3   Is the biomedical paradigm being extended or questioned?

As a result of this construction of trauma, am I more or less likely to focus on the "symptoms" and limitations of women who have experienced abuse? How deterministic are the claims about the effects of violence that are being made? When the biological implications of trauma are being discussed, is space for uncertainty being granted? How prescriptive is the treatment or response that is being offered? How rigid is the definition of "recovery" that is being used? Is an individualistic understanding of "recovery" being drawn upon, based upon individual traits or efforts, or is "recovery" and "resilience" understood to stem from social and material resources? Is there space to critique the assumptions and effects of mental health services and practices, including the reality that sometimes accessing mental health services makes things worse rather than better?

4   Is a normative or transformative view of "illness" and "dysfunction" being utilised?

While the claim within some versions of trauma that a person is "unwell, though understandably so" may lead to some improvements in service provision, the legitimacy of notions of "mental illness/ abnormality" and the opposing notion of "mental health" often remain unchallenged within such constructions. Therefore, it is useful to ask: Is this construction of trauma premised upon a categorisation of human experience as either "normal" or "abnormal" ("traumatised")? How are service users being positioned: is the focus merely on "symptom" assessment and alleviation, or is distress viewed as a meaningful and legitimate response to violence, where treatment may not be required or useful? Are notions of "recovery" being defined by service users or by expert professionals? Furthermore, is "recovery" constructed as compulsory and/or essential?

5   Is a bigger-picture analysis of social and political structures made possible?

What actions are being suggested by this version of trauma? Is the focus of the responses based upon providing services at an individual level only, or are suggestions being made about possibilities for activist work or other broader suggestions beyond the level of individuals, including social policy responses and prevention work? Is the term "trauma" being used as a replacement term, or interchangeably, with words including violence, abuse, and inequality? If so, what are the implications for the responses that are being suggested? Does the discussion move beyond a recognition of *social context*, towards a discussion about social justice, power relations, and a commitment to the need for social change?

The slipperiness of the trauma concept is clear: it has been used to justify the need for taking resolute steps to reduce the use of seclusion and restraint within mental health inpatient settings, due to the harm caused by these practices for service users who have already survived other forms of violence (Chandler, 2008). As a result, although the trauma concept is far from a necessary component of a radical critique of psychiatric practices, it has legitimised and boosted human rights perspectives within mental health settings. On other occasions, the trauma paradigm is enacted in a much more generic fashion, for example, to suggest pest-control measures and providing a clean building for service users – recommendations that are unattached to the specificities of violence or oppression, and that could be considered basic requirements for any human service setting (Becker-Blease, 2017). The amorphous quality of the trauma concept means that it can be drawn upon pragmatically within the constraints of the existing mental health system in order to make space for women's voices and feminist activism, however with this opportunity comes the need to exercise vigilance about its multiple uses, especially the erasure of feminist perspectives and analyses of power. A narrow focus on symptom assessment, treatment modalities, and neurobiological processes precludes a myriad of other possibilities for understanding gender-based violence and effectively responding to patriarchal contexts beyond medical and therapeutic contexts.

Alternatives to therapeutic governance

The narratives in Chapter 5 brought into view the value that the participants placed upon therapy as a response to distress following experiences of gender-based violence, even within a context of disappointing or harmful outcomes. The women's narratives are reflective of a broad ideology present within "therapeutic societies" that when troubled, it is useful to talk, and that it is especially beneficial to engage the expert guidance of a helping professional (Moloney, 2013). By definition, all therapeutic approaches involve – to greater or lesser extents – an exploration of service users' biographical and social contexts, in contrast to an entirely de-contextualised biomedical discourse. This obvious improvement is helpful in understanding why therapeutic practices have often escaped the feminist critique that has been so vital in identifying the limitations of other mental health practices. Despite the ability of therapy to locate distress within a broader social milieu in comparison to a medication-only paradigm, there has been a limited analysis within critical mental health literature on the limitations of a therapeutic response to the problem of gender-based violence, due to a focus on critiquing medication-based and diagnostic practices.

The ambivalence that the participants expressed towards therapeutic interventions occurred within a context of limited options and a sense of personal responsibility for engaging in processes of self-management following experiences of violence. Their mixed and seemingly contradictory thoughts on therapy reflect Kelly and Chapman's (2015, p. 46) disconcerting analysis of the hidden power relations within human service interactions:

> [S]ociety is arranged in such a way that professional services are indispensable for many to survive, and service users can experience them as simultaneously helpful and oppressive.

Although perhaps too quick to dismiss therapy outright and the complex and understandable reasons why people may access therapeutic support in neoliberal contexts that offer few other avenues for support, Furedi helpfully critiques the prominence of emotional wellbeing discourses within psychocentric societies. The pursuit of happiness despite adversities is a goal that is mediated through professional therapeutic expertise:

> Intrusion into the world of people's thinking has become institutionalised under the present system of evolving therapeutic governance. There is very little opposition to this trend and hardly any concern with the potentially authoritarian implications of . . . telling people how to feel.
>
> (Furedi, 2004, p. 64)

Trauma therapies are not homogenous, and contemporary trauma literature is replete with attempts to determine the most efficacious therapeutic modalities and to differentiate between trauma treatments, with trauma-focused cognitive behavioural therapy combining trauma principles with already highly influential cognitive approaches (J. A. Cohen, Mannarino, & Deblinger, 2012), while a range of sensory-based, somatic, and expressive therapies are gaining increased prominence (Steele & Malchiodi, 2012). Dialectical Behaviour Therapy (DBT), developed for Borderline Personality Disorder, offers another influential approach that integrates cognitive methods with emotion-focused strategies including acceptance and meditation (Enns, 2003). While DBT is widely considered to be highly efficacious in reducing suicidal behaviour and inpatient admissions, the majority of research has been conducted within tightly controlled research lab settings (Carmel, Rose, & Fruzzetti, 2014). Recently, the promising results of eye movement desensitisation and reprocessing (EMDR) and neuro feedback strategies have also gained prominence (van der Kolk, 2014). However, it is unclear whether the reported success of EMDR is related specifically to the eye movements that it specifies, or simply the more general elements that it shares with a traditional cognitive approach (Anastas, 2012).

At a broader level, debates about the most efficacious therapeutic techniques for trauma provide a distraction from the similarities shared by many trauma therapies. While trauma therapies provide contextualised understandings of service users' "symptoms", locating distress as a meaningful and understandable response to violence or other adverse events, they frequently continue to assess service users for signs of abnormal perceptions and behaviours, for example, by assessing for "learned fear responses" (J. Cohen, Mannarino, & Murray, 2011), and to emphasise the need for individual processes of adaptation. In this way, many trauma therapies are based upon locating problems within the belief systems of service users, with the person who has survived violence being situated as the target of change. Also, the focus on therapeutic efficacy sidesteps a broader discussion about the limitations of therapy in both preventing and responding to gender-based violence, and important questions about the professional and financial interests that are entwined within the development of "new" therapies, inventories, and treatment modalities.

Nevertheless, as described in Chapter 3, some forms of therapy do manage to engage with social justice issues, offering women the opportunity to locate their distress within its broader social milieu, and to discuss structural inequalities rather than focusing on individual change processes. Due to the individualising effects of mainstream therapeutic practices, mental health workers engaging in trauma work may reject cognitive approaches to therapy based on changing the belief systems of service users and attempt instead to engage in more politicised work (see Tseris, 2018), and Chapter 3 outlined the important contributions of feminist and other critical approaches to therapy. The development of a critical awareness of the limited capacities of therapy, then, is not the same as arguing that therapy is never useful to women, and it is crucial to examine the ways in which narratives that are developed within therapeutic contexts have the capacity to play a powerful role in denouncing atrocities and demanding justice (Herrero, 2015). While cognitive and critical approaches in therapy share the goal of making changes to the ways that service users are viewing their experiences, critical and feminist paradigms do so on a much larger scale, where the emphasis is re-positioned from the self to society, potentially opening up ways of responding to gender-based violence that move beyond fixing individual service users. Such practices are useful in bridging the unhelpful divide that sometimes exists between structural analysis and the lived and felt experience of inequality (Robinson, 2011), and in examining the covert ways in which feminists may endeavour to enact social change within the constraints of existing mental health systems.

Despite these improvements to mainstream therapeutic practices, however, a broader critique of the central positioning of therapy as a response to gender-based violence is also desperately required, particularly as the trauma paradigm becomes increasingly focused on an individual treatment approach. Taking a more measured approach to understanding the benefits of therapy can enable therapy to be re-positioned from a "common-sense" pathway following violence to merely one possible response among many. Developing a healthy scepticism about the limited capacities of psychiatric discourses, therapy, and the trauma paradigm, in assisting women with experiences of gendered oppression can lead to a broader examination of the socio-political causes and consequences of women's distress, which sit outside of an individual's biological or psychological make-up.

Exploring social justice outcomes

Social justice rhetoric is becoming ubiquitous within social work and related professions. At the same time, human service workers are being asked to demonstrate the efficacy of their work within neoliberal contexts that privilege clinical interventions based upon modifying the beliefs and behaviours of service users, in contrast to systemic advocacy work (Kam, 2014). Of concern, while human service education includes social justice aspirations, questions relating to how such values might be enacted within the day-to-day work within agency contexts have exposed complexities and contradictions within human service work (Bhuyan, Bejan, & Jeyapal, 2017). Such contradictions are evident within the growing emphasis on an individualised trauma paradigm that focuses on women's psychological deficiencies, diverting attention away from important discussions about how women might experience just outcomes following violence. In the midst of the contemporary turn towards trauma as a response to gender-based violence, it is worthwhile giving consideration to questions about what is currently *not* being discussed and addressed within mainstream trauma discourses, what options are being denied to women, and the interests that are served by these silences. In addition to a determination to improve the therapy that is available for women who have experienced violence, the community ideologies that support the perpetration of gender-based violence and that continue to create extremely hostile contexts for women who seek support and justice must also be targeted. Such analyses could extend beyond the well-documented constraints of the legal system as a response to gender-based violence and towards much broader questions about how the conditions that allow violence to occur might be addressed (Howe, 2018). Access to safety and material resources, including safe, affordable housing is pivotal to women's capacity to establish a life free from abuse, without which it is arguably impossible to engage in "recovery" of any kind (Hetling, Dunford, Lin, & Michaelis, 2018). Although these ideas may appear to be self-evident, the current construction of trauma-informed perspectives as a "game changer" (Weinhold & Weinhold, 2018), both within mental health settings and human service contexts more generally, has centralised a treatment response and this dominant positioning affects the attention, time, and resources that are able to be given to more systemic approaches to gender equality, including refuges, law reform, and income security – efforts that were pivotal to second-wave feminist activist work. The need to protect these resources is ever more pressing within contemporary neoliberal contexts, keeping in mind that women, and in particular, marginalised women are disproportionately affected by austerity measures (Pruitt, Hamilton, Heydon, & Spark, 2017), and professional therapeutic responses can do little to address widening social inequalities.

There are, concurrently, reasons to be concerned about the social justice impli-cations of doing away altogether with the trauma paradigm. Notably, the rele-vance of the trauma concept has been challenged not only by critical and feminist voices but also by those wishing to question the legitimacy of women in speaking out about the existence and effects of gendered oppression. Such perspectives have sought to describe feminists and other advocates for women and children's rights as enacting a "victimological paradigm" that has exaggerated the extent and impacts of abuse (Oellerich, 2000, p. 71). Such perspectives play neatly into the hands of neoliberal mental health discourses, which are characterised not only by both coercive practices, as described in Chapter 2, but also neglect and the denial of attention or resources (Sawyer, 2008) – for example, through offering only brief support based upon notions of self-management and personal responsibility (Martin, 2013). Within such contexts, service users who are unable to thrive or "recover" risk being classed "non-compliant" or "treatment resistant", rather than as an indication of a mental health system that promises remarkable cures but frequently fails to provide meaningful support. As the majority of the "symptoms" that women present with following violence are likely to remain intractable when addressed only through biomedical means (Long, 2011), women are particularly vulnerable to being placed in the category of an "unmotivated" service user. It is important, then, to note the ways in which critical perspectives on trauma risk being co-opted by a neoliberal mental health policy agenda in order to provide renewed justifications for a low tolerance of women's distress. A social justice approach to trauma, then, must explore both the hazards of pathologising women and enacting unwanted mental health interventions that medicalise women's experiences, while at the same time avoiding a cruel detachment from the imme-diate needs of women in distress.

As trauma-informed perspectives offer a strategy for articulating and defending against inequalities, feminist scholars and human service workers cannot afford to entirely reject them, however a more careful analysis of the trauma paradigm's multiple meanings and implications is needed. In response to this challenge, I would like to suggest the need for a *de-therapising* approach to trauma, which utilises the benefits of the trauma paradigm in harnessing a recognition of the problem of violence against women, but that privileges socio-political questions and is vigilant regarding the co-option and watering down of feminist work within mental health services. Engagement with a de-therapising agenda would involve extending the trauma concept beyond the modest aspiration of "fine-tuning" men-tal health services, while ultimately leaving their core assumptions and practices intact. Instead, it would consider how it might be possible to find ways of engag-ing with women's distress outside of the confines of medicalised and therapeutic support, as well as addressing questions relating to violence prevention and social change. Such work would draw upon and expand the important contributions of feminist therapy's dual engagement with the material realities of women's distress and an ambitious social change agenda. Examples include community activism and political engagement (Weldon & Htun, 2013), policy interventions (Michau, Horn, Bank, Dutt, & Zimmerman, 2014), groupwork education and prevention

(Ball et al., 2012), and strengthening peer support (Tajima, Herrenkohl, Moylan, & Derr, 2011). As argued by Bracken (in Hall, 2016, pp. 230–231), therapy fails to offer a background context in which suffering can be fully understood:

> [S]ome good individual and counselling work can be done, but meaningfulness is about our actual connection to one another . . . that can happen through all sorts of things: faith, religion, art, creativity, politics, sport, and community activism. There's a whole series of routes.

Critical explorations of therapy, such as in the study reported on in Chapter 5 outlining women's complex negotiations of professional mental health discourses, are helpful in disturbing the perceived centrality of a therapeutic response to women's distress following violence. This empirical research complements a sociological critique of the limitations of therapy that was outlined in Chapter 3. The participants' vexed engagements with medicalised and therapeutic discourses draw attention to the need for research into the aftermath of gender-based violence that is not merely focused on symptom and "treatment" issues or the measurement of therapeutic efficacy, but that examines the pathways of women who have navigated the aftermath of gender-based violence through means other than individualised medical or therapeutic support. A de-therapising agenda can challenge psychocentric thinking about violence and its effects – while also keeping in mind the pitfalls of neoliberal thinking about the triviality of women's despair, and an individualised resilience agenda that places the burden squarely upon women to manage the effects of violence as isolated individuals. A de-therapising approach to trauma is useful in differentiating between lived experiences of violence and the explanatory frameworks provided by trauma discourses, and in providing expanded ways of thinking about how support, connection, skill-building, education, resources, and opportunities following violence can be provided to women outside of the constraints of therapeutic agenda focused on individual change and adaptation. At the same time, acknowledging the lack of such opportunities for many women following experiences of gender-based violence can provide nuanced explanations relating to why women might continue to access therapy in the midst of disappointing outcomes, thus avoiding situating women as hapless recipients of therapeutic discourses.

Caution relating to new sites of trauma

In Chapter 3, I discussed proposals relating to the inclusion of additional trauma-based disorders into the DSM, for example, Complex Post-traumatic Stress Disorder (C-PTSD) or Developmental Trauma Disorder (Van der Kolk, 2017) – advocacy efforts that are based upon concerns that PTSD is the only diagnosis that incorporates a recognition of the role of life events in the development of human distress, and that it does not adequately describe the effects of recurrent, interpersonal experiences of violence or abuse. Given the large number of new diagnoses that were incorporated into the DSM-5, it is worth reflecting on the political conditions that led to the DSM-5 not incorporating these categories relating to trauma, and how this connects to psychiatry's historical and ongoing denial of the pervasiveness of gender-based violence and its role in shaping women's experiences of distress. Nevertheless, the attempt by trauma advocates to advance women and children's rights by expanding an already excessively large DSM is concerning. It contrasts with feminism's role in critiquing diagnoses and psychiatric discourses, by ultimately increasing the perceived utility and legitimacy of the DSM. The need to include complex or developmental trauma diagnoses in the DSM has been justified on the basis that:

> This condition is rampant in foster, adopted as well as kinship care populations, and particularly in First Nation populations . . . as are the accompanying severe attachment disorders and the full array of diverse learning, behavioral, and emotional co-morbidity.
>
> (Bremness & Polzin, 2014, p. 144)

In this short description, it is clear that any new trauma diagnoses will reinforce psychiatry's bias towards labelling already marginalised groups of people as dysfunctional and in need to "fixing" rather than addressing structural inequalities, creating new markets for expert interventions, and re-casting the effects of violence and racism as evidence of mental illness, in order to justify further social control in the form of psychiatric assessments. This reflects the ways in which activist and service user led understandings ("recovery", "empowerment", and so on) have been, time and again, incorporated into mental health policy and practice contexts with hopes about their capacity to create system changes, only to be watered down and re-interpreted according to conventional psychiatric practices (Penney & Prescott, 2016). Therefore, despite the new category of *Trauma and Stressor Related Disorders* in the DSM, which does recognise the role of external events in shaping distress, the expansion of the DSM to incorporate yet more diagnoses is hazardous. As a result, while advocacy regarding the DSM may be successful in garnering social attention toward the problem of violence against women and children by positioning it as a serious issue that is linked to major mental distress, it may act as a distraction from a myriad of other potential social actions that are important in responding to violence against women and children outside of the constraints of the mental health system. Further, it may expose women to further stressors and modes of control, in the form of unwanted interventions and psychiatric surveillance.

Although not the focus of this book, a proliferation of trauma discourses is also evident in a range of contexts beyond women's mental health and gender-based violence. The development of specific trauma diagnoses and treatment protocols has been presented as a necessary step in effectively understanding and responding to the effects of global crises, atrocities, and disasters, for example, the establishment of trauma-informed services to understand and support the needs of refugees and asylum seekers. This has raised substantial concerns about the underpinning assumption that mental health discourses are universally relevant and culturally transferable. As Furedi (2014, p. 15) warns, "when Western therapeutic ideals are projected internationally, they risk pathologizing the people who are offered recognition". In the same way that therapeutic responses to gender-based violence tend to construct women's distress following violence as problematic and requiring intervention, trauma discourses enacted in other contexts risk utilising a similarly de-contextualised and pathologising understanding of violence and its effects. The utilisation of a trauma perspective and a therapeutic approach to managing distress in contexts of ongoing conflict and uncertainty has been critiqued for the assumption that it is reasonable to expect people to adapt to and accept injustice and prolonged uncertainty (Marshall, 2014). The trauma paradigm is also involved in elevating and imposing Western understandings, and concealing or – worse still – jeopardising local coping strategies (Pupavac, 2001). At the same time, the trauma paradigm has played an enormously important role in disrupting societal indifference towards humanitarian crises, and it is therefore understandable that activists have drawn upon the trauma concept to draw attention to otherwise invisibilised suffering, violence, and human rights violations (Service for the Treatment and Rehabilitation of Torture and Trauma Survivors, 2016). There is a tension, then, between the necessity of drawing upon the trauma paradigm in an attempt to mobilise social action, and the need to critique its individualising and pathologising effects. When negotiating these complexities, attention must be given to enacting a more expansive view on trauma than is provided by the DSM, including addressing crucial questions about how to promote southern expertise rather than merely imposing pre-determined diagnostic categories (Johnson, 2012).

Another emergent site of trauma is found in the concept of "vicarious trauma" (also known as compassion fatigue, secondary traumatisation, or burnout), which is understood to be the trauma experienced by human service workers as a result of the emotional toll of working with survivors of violence (Richardson, in National Sexual Violence Resource Center, 2013, p. 46). In order to reduce their own risk of developing trauma symptoms, workers are encouraged to engage in a range of self-care strategies, including supervision and debriefing, exercise, spending time with family, attending training workshops to learn skills in protecting their mental health, or even participating in therapy themselves (Kanno & Giddings, 2017). The focus of vicarious trauma discourses on identifying and addressing symptoms within individual workers mirrors many of the limitations of the trauma paradigm and its implications for service users. Without denying the material reality of distress, Reynolds (2011, pp. 28–29) queries the ways in which notions of vicarious trauma position workers who are distressed as deficient, ignoring the socio-political conditions of human service work in contexts of violence and inequality:

> I do not deny that as therapists and community workers we can be harmed and experience pain in our work, even to the extent of needing to leave the work, or take time out. What I am contesting is the prescriptive, individualised accusations burnout levies against workers which invisibilise and obscure the contexts of social injustice we work in, and blame clients for the harms we experience.

Indeed, Morrison (2007) notes that time spent working with survivors of violence is the best predictor of trauma scores among therapists, and that it is little coincidence that therapists with a higher percentage of sexual assault survivors in their caseload report more PTSD symptoms. Too much emphasis on worker behaviours within the vicarious trauma literature ignores the need for organisational support, and invokes an assumption that the inherently upsetting nature of working with violence can be side-stepped through behavioural strategies. Therefore, while the use of trauma discourses to describe workers' distress is useful in acknowledging the difficulty of their work and the strategies that may be necessary to manage the effects of witnessing the pain of others (Penny, 2016), it may not adequately account for effects of the unjust and under-resourced contexts of human services work. Instead, a narrow view on vicarious trauma risks positioning workers' distress as evidence of inadequate self-care or – worse still – an inappropriate reaction to witnessing injustice, justifying the need for a mental health intervention. Additionally, as Reynolds notes in the quotation above, service users are at risk of being blamed as the cause of workers' distress.

Feminism in mental health

Given the now extensive breadth of feminist critiques of psychiatric interventions (Burstow, 2003; Ussher, 2011), it is time for feminist perspectives to be taken seriously within mental health contexts, so that the responses that are provided – whether or not service users have disclosed an experience of abuse or violence – are informed by understandings of how unequal power and gendered oppression affect the everyday lives of women. When these links are not made, women's distress risks being re-interpreted through the lens of conventional psychiatry – at best, leading to a label of trauma, resulting in a potential array of complicated implications that have been outlined in this book – but often also leading to more pejorative labels, including Borderline Personality Disorder (BPD). Although discussions about gender and mental health are increasing commonplace, they are often incomplete. For example, discussions relating to women's overrepresentation in the mental health system often minimise gendered stressors in the development of distress that is labelled as mental illness (Moulding, 2015). Instead, research commonly explores women's higher propensity for help-seeking behaviours, the stoicism of men, and practitioners' lack of knowledge pertaining to indicators of distress in men (Möller-Leimkühler, 2002). Leaving aside the problem that discussions of this kind are premised upon outdated notions of a binary distinction between the experiences and behaviours of men and women, such explanations assume that the mental health services being provided to women are helpful, when the vast majority of mental health support that is provided to women is oriented towards symptom management, is decontextualised from women's social worlds, and is devoid of an analysis of gendered power relations. Therefore, women may come under the gaze of psychiatric services more frequently than men, but this is not necessarily to their advantage (Ussher, 2018). As I have argued, even trauma-informed paradigms frequently rely on notions of symptom management and thus are not necessarily to women's advantage, as they do not necessarily incorporate feminist knowledge about women's experiences of violence.

Language is important, too: "including – maybe even *particularly* – language that seems innocuous" (Burstow, 2013, p. 90). As mental health discourse shifts towards a trauma paradigm, and service user experiences are increasingly viewed through the lens of trauma, there is a risk that more accurate descriptors of gender-based violence and other structural oppressions and inequalities are being lost. Chapter 4 explored how the trauma concept is increasingly used as a blanket term to describe experiences as wide-ranging as poverty, bullying, divorce, and car accidents, with some writers claiming that trauma is "a fact of life" (Levine, 1997, p. 2). The genericising of trauma is reducing the capacity of the trauma paradigm to address the specific power relations, social contexts, and community responses that are relevant to different types of adverse life events. In considering gender-based violence specifically, it is notable how often the term "trauma" is used in human services literature as a replacement term for words including violence, sexual assault, gender inequality, rape, and abuse, thus leading to the sanitising of women's experiences of violence. Unpacking the ways in which language usage in mental health settings elevates particular perspectives and invisibilises others illuminates the inherently political nature of all mental health work (Tseris, 2016). When human service workers comment that women who have experienced abuse and violence "have PTSD and need to go to therapy to address their trauma", they are often not intending to enact oppressive or coercive practices. Yet, there is an urgent need to examine the assumptions that underpin the notion of a "trauma-tised" woman, and for critical thinking relating to questions including: What do we mean by "trauma"? Are there other ways of viewing what has occurred? Is it the case that women are uniformly affected by violence in predictable ways? In what ways does the phrase "addressing trauma" place responsibility for abuse on survivors rather than perpetrators or broader societal structures? To what extent does the reprocessing of memories assist in enabling women to live meaning-ful adult lives? Will therapy produce the same outcomes for all women? How would we determine whether the therapy has "worked"? What happens when therapy "doesn't work"? Where does the notion of social justice fit in with these discussions?

In addition, feminist theory's attention to gender inequality and gendered role expectations is relevant not only when providing mental health interventions to women, but also to the mental health support provided to people of other genders across a variety of contexts. For example, mental health work with men can be enhanced by a feminist analysis that illuminates how men are adversely affected by rigid scripts of masculinity, despite experiencing other aspects of masculine privilege (Alston, 2012). A feminist analysis is also pertinent when supporting men who have survived interpersonal violence, in recognising that the majority of violence experienced by boys and men has been perpetrated by men (Taft, Hegarty, & Flood, 2001). Beyond this, however, Moulding (2017) invites human service workers to consider how gender stereotypes may be implicit within the sup-ports that are typically provided to men who have been identified as traumatised.

For example, she discusses the need for the responses provided to men following childhood abuse to actively critique rigid and limiting constructions of masculinity (for instance, ideas that the effects of abuse can be managed through becoming a "strong man" who is in control of his emotions). Such analyses highlight the ways in which patriarchal relations diminish the lives of people of all genders, reflecting hooks' (2000) contention that "feminism is for everybody".

Concluding reflections

The value of critical analysis is sometimes challenged on the basis that it involves the breaking down of commonly accepted truths about the social world, while at the same time failing to offer alternative ways forward. On the other hand, critical theorists have lamented the turn in mental health activism from an anti-psychiatry perspective towards a less radical, reformist attempt to work with mental health professionals towards changing – rather than dismantling – the mental health system (Esposito & Perez, 2014). My hope in writing this book is that the pitfall of pessimistic critique has been avoided, through the book's recognition that feminist efforts have been enacted from within the constraints of psychiatric service systems, while at the same time noting the pressing need for feminist action to continue to occur beyond the bounds of mental health contexts. The analysis offered in this book has tried to straddle the competing demands of offering a sharp critique of the contemporary uptake of trauma, while also recognising that the trauma paradigm has made a difference to some women's experiences of mental health services. I concur with the sentiment put forward by Foote and Frank (1999, p. 157), whereby in their critical appraisal of grief counselling, they argue for tentativeness about mental health work, which nonetheless avoids descending into paralysis:

> Our point is not to render therapy impossible but to extend therapists' sense of how problematic their work is.

In contrast to a construction of therapeutic work that accepts comforting narratives about benevolence and empowerment, a critical and de-therapised view on trauma might enable workers to become more curious about the limitations of their practices and the hidden power relations that are embedded within every therapeutic encounter, and most definitely to avoid the temptation to simply say that "more" or "better" therapy is needed. Instead, a de-therapisation approach might explore responses to violence that can occur outside of the confines of therapy, while also noting that the integration of feminist theory into therapeutic practices is possible, though difficult. A critical posture also engages with the utility of trauma discourses in speaking back to notions of individual responsibility that are embedded within neoliberal ideologies, which minimise women's experiences of distress. At the same time, Chapter 5 demonstrated the limitations of such advocacy, given that trauma paradigm also risks positioning women as personally responsible for resolving their emotional distress and re-engaging in productive and optimistic forms of personhood. If the trauma concept is to be utilised, then, it is important that this occurs in a way that is attentive to its mixed and some-times unintended effects, including its propensity to re-direct the responsibili-ties for managing social issues onto individuals or to re-inscribe long-standing practices of labelling women as mentally deficient. In considering the multiple effects of the popularisation of trauma discourses within mental health settings, it may be useful to take Stanley Cohen's (1998, p. 112) pragmatic advice, strategi-cally drawing upon the trauma concept where useful, but also being aware of its capacity to conceal inequalities and to inhibit social change processes through the elevation of therapeutic expertise:

> Stay in your agency or organisation, but do not let it seduce you. Take every opportunity to unmask its pretensions and euphemisms, use its resources in a defensive way for your clients, work for abolition.

Of course, whenever trauma-informed practices lead to more compassionate men-tal health service provision, in which reaching for a biochemical or hormonal explanation for women's distress is replaced with a recognition of the role played by gender injustices on women's lives, this step forward must be celebrated. The popularisation of the trauma paradigm means that gender-based violence has been rendered "thinkable" (Fullagar, 2009) within mental health settings, and this is no small achievement. The trauma concept has provided a means through which pre-viously silenced conversations about social justice within mental health settings have been able to commence, though imperfectly and often with double-edged consequences.

In addition to its incisive analysis of power relations, an important contribu-tion of critical mental health theory is an attention to intersections and multiplici-ties. In a first-person account, Rachel Waddingham (2017, p. 189) discusses the inability of a trauma narrative to explain the origins of her experiences of hearing voices and paranoia (terms that she describes as inadequate, instead choosing the term "toxicity"):

> I hate the idea that the things that happened to me as a child define such a deep and pervasive part of me. I no longer want to identify as a victim, and even seeing myself as a survivor almost prioritises the actions of others in what I have become. It's as if the beautiful and warm parts of my childhood are obscured by those in which I was overwhelmed. I cannot disown or deny the impact my formative years had on my identity, yet I want to look beyond this. I refuse to frame my toxicity as a pathological part of myself that is an understandable consequence of childhood abuse. That is not the story I wish to carry forwards into my life. I need another one.

Waddingham's powerful narrative challenges the singular trauma narrative, instead highlighting the involvement of trauma discourses in the creation of new exclusions, marginalisations, and hierarchies of knowledge production within mental health settings. Therefore, when mental health workers espouse the capacity of the trauma concept to achieve feminist and social justice aims, space and attention is also needed for different explanatory frameworks and diverse experiences. The narratives documented in Chapter 5 included an array of pathways after violence that did not fit within narrow diagnostic and therapeutic expectations, and women were appreciative of workers who were able to act responsively rather than prescriptively. Reflecting complexities in feminist practices, and the tensions between second-wave and poststructural feminism that were discussed in Chapter 2, Mohanty (2003, p. 2) claims that "our most expansive and inclusive visions of feminism need to be attentive to borders while learning to transcend them". Here, she implies that while the "borders" of language and categorisation enable spaces of activism to be carved out, such processes become problematic when attempting to "settle on" a universal concept of women's suffering.

The trauma paradigm must not become the new "truth" of women's mental health experiences, replacing the rigidities of biomedical reductionism with newfound certainties, or – more troubling still – using different words to continue to perpetuate the core assumptions of biomedical psychiatry. It is necessary to resist the positioning of trauma theory as a panacea for women's mental health, and to develop some clarity about its inability to fully address the origins of women's distress. In addition to its socially transformative capacity, the trauma paradigm can be used to reflect and perpetuate the dominant norms and power relations of neoliberal and patriarchal societies, in the forms of diagnosis, normative notions of "recovery", and self-monitoring and responsibilisation discourses. As trauma-informed practices primarily exert their influence at the levels of individual workers and mental health service systems, it is important to acknowledge that substantial energy and resources are also required to develop broader political and social responses to address and eliminate the problem of gender-based violence. It is my hope that this book provides a small contribution to this ongoing work.

References

Alston, M. (2012). Rural male suicide in Australia. *Social Science & Medicine*, *74*(4), 515–522.

Anastas, J. W. (2012). From scientism to science: How contemporary epistemology can inform practice research. *Clinical Social Work Journal*, *40*(2), 157–165.

Ball, B., Tharp, A. T., Noonan, R. K., Valle, L. A., Hamburger, M. E., & Rosenbluth, B. (2012). Expect respect support groups: Preliminary evaluation of a dating violence prevention program for at-risk youth. *Violence Against Women*, *18*(7), 746–762.

Becker-Blease, K. A. (2017). As the world becomes trauma-informed, work to do. *Journal of Trauma & Dissociation*, *18*(2), 131–138.

Bhuyan, R., Bejan, R., & Jeyapal, D. (2017). Social workers' perspectives on social justice in social work education: When mainstreaming social justice masks structural inequalities. *Social Work Education*, *36*(4), 373–390.

Bremness, A., & Polzin, W. (2014). Commentary: Developmental trauma disorder: A missed opportunity in DSM V. *Journal of the Canadian Academy of Child and Adolescent Psychiatry*, *23*(2), 142–145.

Burstow, B. (2003). Toward a radical understanding of trauma and trauma work. *Violence Against Women, 9*(11), 1293–1317.

Burstow, B. (2013). A rose by any other name: Naming and the battle against psychiatry. In B. A. LeFrancois, R. J. Menzies, & G. Reaume (Eds.), *Mad matters: A critical reader in Canadian mad studies* (pp. 79–90). Toronto: Canadian Scholars' Press.

Carmel, A., Rose, M. L., & Fruzzetti, A. E. (2014). Barriers and solutions to implementing dialectical behavior therapy in a public behavioral health system. *Administration and Policy in Mental Health and Mental Health Services Research, 41*(5), 608–614.

Chandler, G. (2008). From traditional inpatient to trauma-informed treatment: Transferring control from staff to patient. *Journal of the American Psychiatric Nurses Association, 14*(5), 363–371.

Cohen, J. A., Mannarino, A. P., & Murray, L. P. (2011). Trauma-focused CBT for youth who experience ongoing traumas. *Child Abuse & Neglect, 35*(8), 637–646.

Cohen, J. A., Mannarino, A. P., & Deblinger, E. (2012). *Trauma focused CBT for children and adolescents: Treatment applications.* New York: The Guildford Press.

Cohen, S. (1998). *Against criminology.* Abigdon & New York: Routledge.

Enns, C. Z. (2003). Contemporary adaptations of traditional approaches to the counseling of women. In M. Kopala & M. Keitel (Eds.), *Handbook of counseling women* (pp. 3–21). Thousand Oaks: Sage.

Esposito, L., & Perez, F. M. (2014). Neoliberalism and the commodification of mental health. *Humanity and Society, 38*(4), 414–442.

Foote, C. E., & Frank, A. W. (1999). Foucault and therapy: The disciplining of grief. In A. S. Chambon, A. Irving, & L. Epstein (Eds.), *Reading Foucault for social work* (pp. 157–188). New York: Columbia University Press.

Fullagar, S. (2009). Negotiating the neurochemical self: Anti-depressant consumption in women's recovery from depression. *Health: An Interdisciplinary Journal for the Social Study of Health, Illness and Medicine, 13*(3), 389–406.

Furedi, F. (2004). *Therapy culture: Cultivating vulnerability in an uncertain age.* London: Routledge.

Furedi, F. (2014). Is it justice? Therapeutic history and the politics of recognition. In E. Speed, J. Moncrieff, & M. Rapley (Eds.), *De-medicalizing misery II* (pp. 1–18). London: Palgrave Macmillan.

Hall, W. (2016). *Outside mental health: Voices and visions of madness.* United States: Madness Radio.

Herrero, D. (2015). Oranges and sunshine: The story of a traumatic encounter. *Humanities, 4*(4), 714–725.

Hetling, A., Dunford, A., Lin, S., & Michaelis, E. (2018). Long-term housing and intimate partner violence: Journeys to healing. *Affilia, online first.* Retrieved from https://doi.org/10.1177/0886109918778064.

hooks, b. (2000). *Feminism is for everybody.* Cambridge: South End Press.

Howe, R. (2018). Community-led sexual violence and prevention work: Utilising a transformative justice framework. *Social Work and Policy Studies: Social Justice, Practice and Theory, 1,* 001.

Johnson, K. (2012). Global mental health, cultural specificity and the risk of neocolonialism: Challenges for critical community psychology. In C. Walker, K. Johnson, & L. Cunningham (Eds.), *Community psychology and the socio-economics of mental distress: International perspectives* (pp. 269–284). Houndmills: Palgrave Macmillan.

Kam, P. K. (2014). Back to the 'social' of social work: Reviving the social work profession's contribution to the promotion of social justice. *International Social Work, 57*(6), 723–740.

Kanno, H., & Giddings, M. M. (2017). Hidden trauma victims: Understanding and preventing traumatic stress in mental health professionals. *Social Work in Mental Health,* *15*(3), 331–353.

Kelly, C., & Chapman, C. (2015). Adversarial allies: Care, harm, and resistance in the helping professions. *Journal of Progressive Human Services, 26*(1), 46–66.

Levine, P. (1997). *Waking the tiger: Healing trauma.* Berkeley: North Atlantic Books.

Long, V. (2011). 'Often there is a good deal to be done, but socially rather than medically': The psychiatric social worker as social therapist, 1945–70. *Medical History, 55*(2), 223–239.

Marshall, D. J. (2014). Save (us from) the children: Trauma, Palestinian childhood, and the production of governable subjects. *Children's Geographies, 12*(3), 281–296.

Martin, J. (2013). Accredited mental health social work in Australia: A reality check. *Australian Social Work, 66*(2), 279–296.

Michau, L., Horn, J., Bank, A., Dutt, M., & Zimmerman, C. (2014). Prevention of violence against women and girls: Lessons from practice. *The Lancet, 385*(9978), 1672–1684.

Mohanty, C. T. (2003). *Feminism without borders: Decolonizing theory, practicing solidarity.* Durham: Duke University Press.

Moloney, P. (2013). *The therapy industry: The irresistible rise of the talking cure, and why it doesn't work.* London: Pluto Press.

Morrison, Z. (2007). *'Feeling heavy': Vicarious trauma and other issues facing those who work in the sexual assault field.* Melbourne: Australian Institute of Family Studies.

Moulding, N. (2015). *Gendered violence, abuse and mental health in everyday lives: Beyond trauma.* London: Routledge.

Moulding, N. (2017). "Becoming a better man": Narrating masculinities after childhood emotional abuse. *Affilia, 33*(1), 39–55.

Möller-Leimkühler, A. M. (2002). Barriers to help-seeking by men: A review of sociocultural and clinical literature with particular reference to depression. *Journal of Affective Disorders, 71*(1–3), 1–9.

National Sexual Violence Resource Center. (2013). *Building cultures of care: A guide for sexual assault services programs.* Retrieved from www.nsvrc.org.

Oellerich, T. D. (2000). Rind, tromovitch, and bauserman: Politically incorrect – Scientifically correct. *Sexuality and Culture, 4*(2), 67–81.

Penney, D., & Prescott, L. (2016). The co-optation of survivor knowledge: The danger of substituted values and voice. In J. Russo & A. Sweeney (Eds.), *Searching for a rose garden: Challenging psychiatry, fostering mad studies.* Monmouth: PCCS Books.

Penny, L. (2016). *Life-hacks of the poor and aimless.* Retrieved from https://thebaffler.com/war-of-nerves/laurie-penny-self-care.

Pruitt, L., Hamilton, G., Heydon, G., & Spark, C. (2017). Abbott's 'budget crisis', CALD women's loss? Service providers explore the impact of funding cuts. *Australian Journal of Political Science, 52*(3), 335–350.

Pupavac, V. (2001). Therapeutic governance: Psycho-social intervention and trauma risk management. *Disasters, 25*(4), 358–372.

Reynolds, V. (2011). Resisting burnout with justice-doing. *International Journal of Narrative Therapy & Community Work, 4,* 27–45.

Robinson, C. (2011). *Beside one's self: Homelessness felt and lived.* Syracuse: Syacuse University Press.

Rose, N. (1999). *Governing the soul.* London: Free Association Books.

Sawyer, A. (2008). Risk and new exclusions in community mental health practice. *Australian Social Work., 61*(4), 327–341.

Service for the Treatment and Rehabilitation of Torture and Trauma Survivors. (2016). *Learn about torture and trauma*. Retrieved from www.startts.org.au/resources/refugees-asylum-seekers-and-trauma/learn-about-torture-and-trauma/.

Steele, W., & Malchiodi, C. A. (2012). *Trauma-informed practices with children and adolescents*. New York: Routledge.

Taft, A., Hegarty, K., & Flood, M. (2001). Are men and women equally violent to intimate partners? *Australian and New Zealand Journal of Public Health, 25*(6), 498–500.

Tajima, E. A., Herrenkohl, T. I., Moylan, C. A., & Derr, A. S. (2011). Moderating the effects of childhood exposure to intimate partner violence: The roles of parenting characteristics and adolescent peer support. *Journal of Research on Adolescence, 21*(2), 376–394.

Tseris, E. (2016). Thinking critically about 'mental health issues' affecting women during/after violence. *Social Alternatives, 35*(4), 37–42.

Tseris, E. (2018). Social work and women's mental health: Does trauma theory provide a useful framework? *British Journal of Social Work, online first. Retrieved from* https://doi.org/10.1093/bjsw/bcy090

Ussher, J. M. (2011). *The madness of women*. East Sussex: Routledge.

Ussher, J. M. (2018). A critical feminist analysis of madness: Pathologising femininity through psychiatric discourse. In B. M. Z. Cohen (Ed.), *Routledge international handbook of critical mental health* (pp. 72–78). London: Routledge.

van der Kolk, B. (2014). *The body keeps the score*. London: Penguin Books.

van der Kolk, B. A. (2017). Developmental trauma disorder: Toward a rational diagnosis for children with complex trauma histories. *Psychiatric Annals, 35*(5), 401–408.

Waddingham, R. (2017). Bad me? Learning from, and living with, toxicity. *Psychosis: Psychological, Social and Integrative Approaches, 9*(2), 187–190.

Weinhold, B. K., & Weinhold, J. B. (2018). *Developmental trauma: The game changer in the mental health profession*. Colorado Springs: CICRCL Press.

Weldon, S. L., & Htun, M. (2013). Feminist mobilisation and progressive policy change: Why governments take action to combat violence against women. *Gender and Development, 21*(2), 231–247.

Index

Acute Stress Disorder 36
Adjustment Disorder 36
Aetiology of Hysteria, The (Freud) 35
American Psychiatric Association (APA)
  8, 15
anti-stigma efforts 20, 21
Anxiety Disorder 23, 36
assessment tools 45–46
attachment disorders 65, 114
attachment theory 66–67

biological sciences 19
biomedical discourse 2–3, 15–16, 48–49,
  59, 107, 111–112
borderline personality disorder (BPD)
  40–42, 109
Brief Trauma Questionnaire (BTQ) 45–46

child abuse 4, 16, 25, 36, 39, 41, 48, 65,
  91, 95, 101
collective trauma 42–43
Community Treatment Orders 18
complex post-traumatic stress disorder
  (C-PTSD), 33, 36, 90, 113
complex trauma 7, 36, 37, 42, 67

"damaged" self 63
developmental trauma 36, 113–114
*Diagnostic and Statistical Manual of
  Mental Disorders* (DSM), 8, 15, 23,
  36–37, 40, 42, 70, 113–115
Dialectical Behaviour Therapy (DBT) 109
disciplinary power 16–17
discourses: biomedical discourses
  2–3, 15–16, 48–49, 59, 107,
  111–112; definition of 5; mental
  health discourses 5–6; neuroscience
  discourses 17, 59–64, 83–84, 100;
  psychiatric discourses 16, 24–26, 52;

risk discourses 70; trauma discourses
  6–7, 32–35, 37, 46, 81–84, 114–115;
  "traumatised mothering" discourse
  64–67
Disinhibited Social Engagement Disorder 36
distress: anti-stigma efforts 20; biomedical
  discourse of 59; development of more
  holistic approaches to understanding
  20; experience of 19; influence of
  social factors 2–3; need for social
  analysis of 18–19; politicised analysis
  of 69; psychiatric diagnoses of 36–37;
  psychosocial approaches 20; social
  theories of 20–21

electroconvulsive therapy (ECT) 39
empowerment 46, 67
essentialism 24
"expert by experience" 10
eye movement desensitisation and
  reprocessing (EMDR) 109

fatherhood 66–67
femininity 40
feminism: intersectional feminism 5; in
  mental health 116–118; poststructural
  approach to 24–26; second-wave
  feminism 4–5, 111; third-wave feminism
  5, 24–26; understanding of 4–5
feminist biologists 19
Foucault, M. 16–17, 26
Freud, S. 23, 35

gender-based violence 4–5, 11, 25, 32, 36,
  41–42, 43–47, 53, 61–62
"global mental health" 22

happiness imperative 52
hegemonic discourses 5–6